STP 1301

Modularity of Orthopedic Implants

Donald E. Marlowe, Jack E. Parr, and Michael B. Mayor, Editors

ASTM Publication Code Number (PCN):
04-013010-54

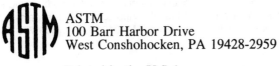

ASTM
100 Barr Harbor Drive
West Conshohocken, PA 19428-2959

Printed in the U.S.A.

ISBN: 0-8031-2415-5
ASTM Publication Code Number (PCN): 04-013010-54

Photocopy Rights

Peer Review Policy

Each paper published in this volume was evaluated by two peer reviewers and at least one editor. The authors addressed all of the reviewers' comments to the satisfaction of both the technical editor(s) and the ASTM Committee on Publications.

To make technical information available as quickly as possible, the peer-reviewed papers in this publication were prepared "camera-ready" as submitted by the authors.

The quality of the papers in this publication reflects not only the obvious efforts of the authors and the technical editor(s), but also the work of these peer reviewers. The ASTM Committee on Publications acknowledges with appreciation their dedication and contribution of time and effort on behalf of ASTM.

Printed in Philadelphia, PA
March 1997

Foreword

This publication, *Modularity of Orthopedic Implants,* contains papers presented at the Symposium on Modularity of Orthopedic Implants held 8 November 1995 in Norfolk, VA. The symposium was sponsored by ASTM Committee F4 on Medical and Surgical Materials and Devices. Donald E. Marlowe, of the FDA Center for Devices and Radiological Health in Rockville, MD; Jack E. Parr, with Wright Medical Technologies in Memphis, TN; and Michael B. Mayor, with the Dartmouth Hitchcock Medical Center in Lebanon, NH, presided as symposium chairmen and are editors of the resulting publication.

Contents

STATE OF THE ART IN PROPERTIES TESTING II

Overview

The assembly of orthopedic prosthetic joint implants from modular components improves the options of the surgeon in the operating room, reduces the inventory of sizes that must be maintained in the hospital and by the manufacturer (distributor), and allows the surgeon to tailor the device to the situation confronted on the operating table. Modularity of implants also presents some interesting problems to the device designer and to the treatment of patients after surgery. In November 1995, ASTM Committee F4, Medical and Surgical Devices and Materials, conducted a symposium on the subject of Modularity of Orthopedic Implants. The objectives of the symposium were to define the knowledge base at the time and provide guidance to the members of the committee who were invested in the development of standards for the measurement of the properties of these devices. The symposium papers published here explore the clinical utility of these devices, the problems presented clinically, and the analytical tools, developed by engineers in manufacturing firms and academic institutions, used to evaluate the devices.

Clinical Relevance

Initially, five papers were scheduled in this session and presented at the symposium. Through several circumstances, only one of these is published in this STP. These authors addressed the rationale, including pros and cons, for using modular design in hip and knee prostheses and in soft tissue attachment using bone anchors. In the only paper of the group published here, Joseph Zuckerman presented a very complete survey of the clinical literature rerlated to total shoulder arthoplasty (TSA) and the introduction of modular designs for TSAs. While acknowledging that the introduction of modular TSAs is relatively new and, therefore, the longevity of the repaired joints is in some question, the early results are very supportive of the modularity concept.

One paper presented as part of this session, but not published in this volume, focused on the general process by which ASTM develops standards. We wish to thank Jack Lemons for sharing his thoughts on the process and mechanics of standards development, and for emphasizing the need for attending the symposium as well as the need for readers of this volume to participate in the development of consenus standards.

Issues of Concern

The issues of concern expressed by the authors of the papers in this session were very wide-ranging. Stuart Goodman reported on a revision series of acetabular components in which no correlation between modularity and the biological indicators of bone remodeling was identified but reported that, at revision surgery, many of the cellular components and cytokines associated with loosening and osteolysis were present. Urban et al. further developed this thought by examining the solid products of corrosion that devlop in modular head-femoral stem joints and expressing concern about the kinetics of these degradation products. Gilbert and Jacobs reviewed several test methods they developed to evaluate mechanically-assisted crevice corrosion and compared test results with corrosion found on retrieved head/stem combinations of several metal alloys. Shea et al. completed the discussion of biological concerns by reporting on the generation of polyethylene particles at the several interfaces in a design of modular acetabular cups. They note that considerable work has been done to control particle generation at the femoral head/acetabular liner interface, but that attention must be paid to reduction of motion at the other interfaces. Finally, Calès noted that understanding and controlling the manufacturing methods of these devices (specifically, marking ceramic femoral heads) is important to ensure that these methods do not contribute to the initiation of failure mechanisms of the arthroplasty device.

State of the Art in Properties Testing

The papers in this session were almost evenly divided between discussions of the mechanical testing of modular devices and discussions of the various corrosion mechanisms that seem to be acting upon them.

Heim reported on a comparative study of the bending fatigue resistance of four modular hip designs. Lambert and McLean developed a method to study the dynamic fixation in torsion of the polymer liner within the acetabular component, and Fosco and Buchanan reported on test methods to study the push-out and lever-out forces of these components. Kirkpatrick studied the static strength of the polymer articulating surface within the tibial tray of modular total knee systems and Anthony reported on a fatigue test for the tibial component. Schmidt described work to assess the raltionship between the impaction force of a ball on a Morse taper stem and the subsequent disassembly forces. Richter studied the relationship between the ductility of the metal stem and the load-carrying capacity of a ceramic ball mated to it. Naesguthe demonstrated the apparent difficulty in manufacturing matching tapers as would be needed to optimize joint load-carrying performance. These papers constitute a starting point for discussion of testing methods for modular hip and knee joints and should be considered by developers of device standards.

Four papers were presented on fretting corrosion mechanisms and aspects of corrosion-testing of modular hip prostheses. The papers by Bhambri et al., Goldberg et al., McLean and Lambert, and Brown et al. present an internally consistent argument for development of a fretting corrosion requirement for these devices. Special attention is given to the mixed-metal couples created by the use of dissimilar alloys in the stem and head of the prosthesis. A considerable body of data is presented with which to begin to define the testing environment, testing frequency, and loading waveform for such a test method.

Significance and Future Work

The symposium showed the clear clinical benefits related to this type of orthopedic joint and identified no new problems with their use that had not been associated with earlier designs of arthoplasty devices. While the magnitudes of some of these corrosion problems remains unquantified and may, at a later date, present a reason to alter the scientific wisdom expressed here, no extreme actions to change current medical practice currently seem justified.

Donald E. Marlowe
Symposium chairman and co-editor;
   FDA, Center for Devices and Radiological Health
   Rockville, MD 20850.

Jack E. Parr
Symposium co-chairman and co-editor;
   Wright Medical Technologies
   Memphis, TN 38002.

Michael B. Mayor
Symposium co-chairman and co-editor;
   Dartmouth Hitchcock Medical Center
   Lebanon, NH 03756.

Clinical Relevance

Joseph D. Zuckerman, [1] Russell J. Cavallo,[2] and Frederick J. Kummer[3]

A REVIEW OF THE USE OF MODULARITY
IN TOTAL SHOULDER ARTHROPLASTY

REFERENCE: Zuckerman, J. D., Cavallo, R.J., and Kummer, F. J., **"A Review of the Use of Modularity in Total Shoulder Arthroplasty,"** *Modularity of Orthopedic Implants, ASTM STP 1301,* Donald E. Marlowe, Jack E. Parr, and Michael B. Mayor, Eds., American Society for Testing and Materials, 1997.

ABSTRACT: Modularity is a recent advance in total shoulder arthroplasty (TSA). The use of a separate head-stem combination permits intraoperative adjustment of soft tissue tension necessary for successful TSA. Modular glenoid components allow auxiliary fixation by various coatings or screws. Short-term clinical results (<5 years) indicate that the results of modular TSA are equivalent to those of monolithic TSA. Several cases of head-stem disassociation have been observed. It is possible that taper corrosion and polyethylene insert failure could occur in the long term, as has been seen with modular hip replacement.

KEYWORDS: modularity, shoulder arthroplasty, humeral prosthesis, glenoid prosthesis

INTRODUCTION

The first shoulder arthroplasty was performed by the French surgeon Pean in 1893 for a proximal humerus destroyed by tuberculosis [1,2]. The modern era of shoulder arthroplasty began in the mid-1950s when Neer published the preliminary results of 12 patients treated with a proximal humeral replacement [3]. Because his results were far superior to resection arthroplasty, he concluded with guarded optimism that the shoulder arthroplasty would wear better than its counterpart in the weight bearing hip. In 1972, Neer and his

[1]Chairman and Chief of Shoulder Surgery, Hospital for Joint Diseases Orthopaedic Institute, 301 East 17th Street, New York, New York, 10003
[2]Resident, Department of Orthopaedic Surgery, Mount Sinai Medical Center, 5 East 98th Street, New York, New York, 10029
[3]Associate Director, Department of Bioengineering, Hospital for Joint Diseases Orthopaedic Institute, 301 East 17th Street, New York, NY, 10003

colleagues designed three different types of fixed-fulcrum prostheses in an effort to eliminate the need for the rotator cuff. The failure of this design was attributed to the increased shear stresses imparted to the glenoid component as a result of the unopposed superior forces produced by deltoid contracture. Other authors confirmed the high rates of mechanical failure with different constrained designs [4-6], and this technique was abandoned.

In 1973, Neer redesigned the humeral prosthesis so that it conformed to the radius of curvature of a newly designed polyethylene glenoid component. This became one of the first nonconstrained total shoulder arthroplasties (TSA). It was designed to (1) limit the amount of bone removed to preserve soft tissue attachments; (2) maintain near-anatomical design to permit the maximum return of motion; (3) avoid mechanical impingement that might lead to mechanical failure; and (4) emphasize the importance of reconstruction of the surrounding soft tissue structures [7]. The success of this implant has been well documented [8,9], but has not deterred the development of alternative prosthetic designs.

Currently, approximately 10,000 shoulder arthroplasties are performed annually in the United States. Despite the fact that this figure has risen exponentially over the years, it remains far less than the half-million total hip and total knee arthroplasties performed annually [10]. Similar to other total joint arthroplasties, replacement of the shoulder can be expected to improve function and dramatically alleviate pain for the vast majority of patients. Early on, however, Neer recognized the shoulder as a unique functional unit, which distinguished it from the hip and knee. The stability of these joints is largely dependent on either the bony congruity or the supporting ligaments, respectively [7]. In the shoulder, however, the shallow glenoid and loose ligamentous support (static stabilizers) provide far less inherent stability but permit much greater range of motion. The supporting musculature (dynamic stabilizers) become critically important for both stability and motion. In fact, the functional success of TSA is largely determined by soft tissue preservation, restoration, and rehabilitation. These considerations make TSA one of the most technically demanding joint replacement procedures performed by the orthopaedic surgeon [2]. More recently, the development of component modularity in TSA has increased the versatility of the implants while at the same time adding new decision-making aspects to the procedure. The purpose of this paper is to provide the recent information on the use of modularity in TSA.

BIOMECHANICS

The glenohumeral joint has the greatest range of motion of all joints in the human body. To achieve this motion, it has evolved with minimal bony constraint. Although the ligaments contribute to limit translation, their contribution to stability is less than in the hip and knee. Stability is provided mainly by the dynamic stabilizers.

Bony architecture in the shoulder affords little inherent stability and in fact may predispose to instability, as conformity and contact area are low relative to other joints. In a cadaveric study by Friedman et al. [31], only 21% of specimens had a congruent relationship between the humeral head and glenoid. In addition, 76% were found to have a humeral head with a smaller radius of curvature than the glenoid. Not only is the radius of curvature different, but the surface area for articulation is markedly dissimilar. The surface area of the humeral head is 2 to 4 times greater than that of the glenoid, and the diameter of the head is nearly twice that of the glenoid [32]. The result is that only a small portion of the humeral head area is in contact with the glenoid fossa at a given time. More importantly, this contact area decreases with certain glenohumeral positions, resulting in a greater force per unit area (stress) across the joint [31,33]. These findings are in contradistinction to those for the hip, where bony congruity is high and is the primary factor for stability. In addition, increased congruity in the hip leads to increased contact area and a more even stress distribution. Studies have determined that the forces across the shoulder are approximately 0.89 times body weight [31], whereas those across the hip are in excess of 3 to 6 times body weight [34]. However, use of the arm with activities of daily living and carrying objects greatly increases these forces [29] and can probably approach those across the hip. This results in higher and more concentrated stresses (force/area) and has implications for TSR longevity, particularly wear and loosening of the glenoid component.

The dynamics of forces acting across the shoulder are also different from those at the hip. Although the position of the glenoid fossa remains relatively constant throughout most of the arc of motion, the shoulder joint does not act strictly as a ball-and-socket articulation. Unlike the hip, at the extremes of motion humeral head rotation is coupled with translation [32]. Studies have found that the rotator cuff is not responsible for these coupled motions and that capsuloligamentous restraints are more likely involved [35]. This again emphasizes the importance of proper soft tissue reconstruction and tensioning in TSA and the potential benefits achieved by a modular design.

HISTORY OF MODULAR JOINT ARTHROPLASTY

The advent of modularity in TSA is a relatively recent event that followed the successful use of modularity in total hip arthroplasty. As expected, there are much more data available on the results of modularity in total hip procedures. For this reason, and because of its applicability to modularity in TSA, we first discuss the relevant issues related to modularity in total hip arthroplasty.

The evolution toward modular prostheses began in 1970, when Harris developed the metal-backed acetabular component [11]. His goal was to replace the bearing insert without disturbing the primary components. The orthopaedic community was slow to accept "modularity," and it was not until the 1980s that modular femoral components became available [12]. These provided a variety of head and neck combinations, which helped reduce hospital inventory while maintaining a broad spectrum of intraoperative versatility [13]. Additional advantages included enhanced exposure during revision operations as a result of modular head removal and the ability to adjust neck length and head diameter for optimal soft tissue tensioning [14,15]. Biomechanically, modularity also provided the opportunity to create improved mixed-alloy systems with different material and mechanical properties. The selection of a rigid, wear-resistant material for the head along with a more flexible material for the stem could offer significant advantages over the use of a single, homogeneous implant [13,16,17]. For example, titanium alloy has been advocated for porous coated uncemented stems because of its relatively low modulus, while cobalt-chrome alloy is favored for the head because of its superior wear properties [18].

The initial success of modular hip prostheses, as defined by the increased versatility, led to the development of additional modularity options. These included the ability independently to size the metaphysis and diaphysis as well as to adjust anteversion. This unfortunately occurred concomitantly with a growing body of evidence of engineering problems with the original modularity options (head-neck interface and two-piece acetabular cup), causing concern that clinical failure could result [19]. It became evident that there were many questions to be answered with respect to the intermediate and long-term performance of modular replacement systems: (1) What is the risk of dissociation of the components? (2) Will micromotion result in mechanical wear (fretting) at the interface? (3) Will corrosion occur at the interface between mixed alloy systems? (4) Will mechanical damage or corrosion increase the risk of long-term failure at the taper connection? and (5) Will mechanical damage or corrosion increase the risk of loosening at the bone-prosthesis or bone-cement interfaces [14]?

The problems associated with modular prostheses can essentially be divided into three categories: (1) structural/engineering; (2) chemical/biological; and (3) technical/intraoperative. In some instances, the concerns are theoretical and have not been linked to clinical failure. The technical problems are the easiest to overcome and simply require careful attention to detail by the surgeon and staff. The surgeon should be responsible for the proper handling of taper components prior to implantation to ensure optimum mechanical integrity and hence clinical performance. Taper interfaces perform better when they are properly cleaned and dried prior to engagement [20,21]. Also, large impact assembly loads optimize locking at the Morse-taper interface [19,22].

The structural/engineering and chemical/biological issues in modular components can be largely addressed with improved quality control standards by manufacturers and better design tolerances to prevent motion at component interfaces [23]. In addition, it has been recommended that modular connections be restricted to areas where bending and torsional loads are not excessive. Design improvements have already been made for acetabular implants with regard to locking strength, polyethylene liner congruency with the metal shell, and polyethylene thickness [19]. Head-neck taper interfaces have been improved by shrink-fit designs that decrease micromotion and fretting and silicone sealants that help prevent ingress of fluid at the taper interface [16].

MODULARITY IN TOTAL SHOULDER ARTHROPLASTY

For many years the most widely used shoulder replacement system was Neer's nonmodular design. With the knowledge gained from early successes with modular total hip arthroplasty, however, the potential benefits of modularity were quickly extended to the area of TSA. The first modular shoulder systems were developed in the mid-1980s for the purpose of enhancing intraoperative versatility and improving visualization during revision procedures [24].

As reports on the long-term results of TSA were published, critical differences with total hip replacement began to emerge. Careful surgical technique for the placement of components and, especially, soft tissue tensioning were clearly linked to the long-term success or failure of TSA. The impact of a deficient rotator cuff (which has no counterpart in the hip) on glenoid component loosening has been reported by many authors [25,26]. Rotator cuff deficiency results in proximal migration and eccentric loading on the superior aspect of the glenoid component. Consequently, a "rocking horse" motion occurs that leads to glenoid loosening. The cited studies and others made it apparent that the success of a TSA was critically dependent on the integrity and balance of the surrounding soft tissue structures [1]. In theory, modular systems enhance the surgeon's ability to optimize soft tissue balancing and function compared with traditional, nonmodular designs. Modularity of the humeral component facilitates soft tissue tensioning and centralization of the humeral head within the rotator cuff [24,27,28]. This, in turn, helps to minimize eccentric loading of the glenoid component, which may ultimately decrease the incidence of glenoid loosening [1]. In addition, optimizing soft tissue tension by modularity also aids in achieving a stable articulation [29,30].

MODULAR SHOULDER DESIGN

Humeral stems can be fabricated from cobalt-chromium alloy or titanium alloy and have a distal cylindrical section with a rectangular proximal section or proximal fins to increase torsional stability within the humeral canal (Fig. 1). Stems can be press-fit, cemented, porous, or coated with hydroxyapatite (HA) for fixation. The taper can be located either on the head or stem (Fig. 2). Placing the taper on the head increases accessibility during surgery and enables designs in which the head can be offset by eccentric taper placement to duplicate normal anatomical orientation (Fig. 3). The taper is smaller than those in THR and has been augmented with adjacent pegs or a separate screw to increase stability (Fig. 4).

Heads are usually cobalt-chromium (one design uses nitrogen implanted titanium alloy) and hemispherical, although at least one design is ellipsoidal. A variety of head radii (typically three) or neck lengths (constant head radius) permits intraoperative soft tissue tensioning. Anteversion can also be designed into the head to increase stability and minimize dislocation in cases with excessive retroversion.

Modular glenoid components consist of an outer metal shell (titanium alloy) with a polyethylene insert (typically three sizes) and were originally developed for cementless fixation—e.g., porous or HA coatings or the use of several screws. Some designs offer several thicknesses of inserts to facilitate soft tissue balance without altering the center of rotation to the extent it would be if accomplished by solely increasing head size. Some

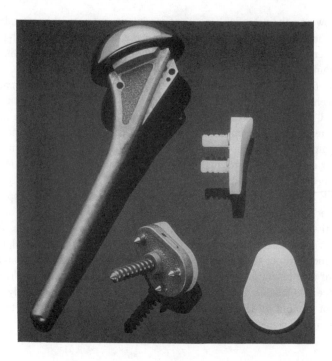

Fig. 1. A typical modular shoulder system. The head is assembled on the humeral shaft; the pad at the top of the stem is for ingrowth fixation. Two alternative glenoid components are shown in side view, one metal-backed and one all-polyethylene; the bearing surface for each is the polyethylene facing shown in lateral view (lower right).

computer modeling studies suggest that an all-polyethylene glenoid component may transfer stress in a more physiologic manner [39]. As a result, surgeons are more inclined to insert nonmodular polyethylene glenoid components in an effort to reduce the risk of glenoid loosening which is the most common cause for a revision complicating TSA.

CLINICAL RESULTS OF MODULAR SHOULDER ARTHROPLASTY

The efficacy of modularity in shoulder arthroplasty must be evaluated in comparison to the clinical results of the nonmodular designs. The most commonly used nonmodular system is the one designed by Neer, and thus many of the clinical results are for the use of this system. Overall, the success rate has been encouraging: over 90% of patients experience good or excellent results in two- to nine-year follow-up [7,9,40]. Pain relief has been reported as excellent in all patient groups undergoing the procedure, but return to function has generally correlated with the integrity of the rotator cuff. It is not surprising, then, that osteoarthritics undergoing TSA have obtained the best functional results

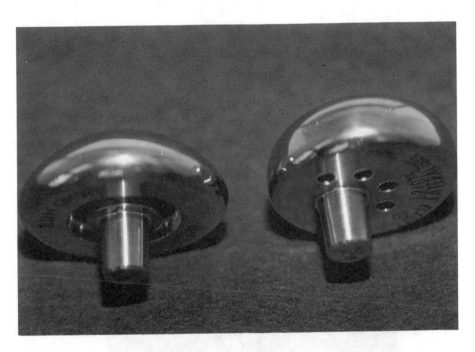

Fig. 2. Offset tapers, which can be used to control head position. (Left) Typical modular head; (right) this head can be "dialed" to the desired degree of numerical translation (the holes on the underside lock with a peg on the humeral stem).

[41]. The rotator cuff in these patients is almost invariably intact, with only 5% of patients having full-thickness tears. Rheumatoid arthritis patients, on the other hand, achieve less dramatic functional gains, since up to 75% will have abnormal rotator cuffs and 20–35% will have full-thickness tears [42].

The clinical results of TSA were recently summarized from 23 series (involving 1459 shoulders) reported from 1982 to 1992 [41]. The incidence of complications was found to be 14% with a minimum two-year follow-up. These included (in order of decreasing frequency): (1) instability (0–22%); (2) rotator cuff tear (1–13%); (3) ectopic ossification (12–40%, rarely clinically significant); (4) glenoid loosening (2% clinical loosening, 30–90% radiolucent lines); (5) intraoperative fracture (<2%); (6) nerve injury (<1%); (7) infection (<1%); and (8) humeral stem loosening (<1%). Implant longevity with nonmodular TSA designs compares favorably with that for total hip arthroplasty patients; revision rates have been approximately 11% at 10 years postoperatively. The most common causes for revision include (1) glenoid loosening; (2) instability; and (3) rotator cuff tearing. These results are from short- and intermediate-range follow-up studies; there are not yet many long-term studies [2]. Torchia et al. [43] reported the results of a series of cases with a mean follow-up of 12.2 years using the Neer prosthesis, found a probability of

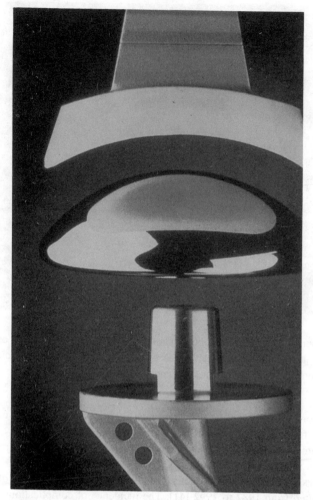

Fig. 3. (Bottom) Tapered male element on humeral stem. (Middle) Head. (Top) Metal-backed polyethylene glenoid component (cement fixation); note curved back in comparison to the flat component in Fig. 1.

implant survival at 15 years of 87%. Relief from moderate or severe pain was achieved in 82% of patients. Of interest were the findings that 84% of patients developed radioluciencies at the bone-cement interface of the glenoid component and that 44% had radiographic evidence of "definite" loosening. The authors concluded that TSA provides reliable long-term pain relief and that, although the glenoid radiolucent lines can progress to radiographic signs of definite loosening, glenoid component revision is only infrequently (5.6%) required [43].

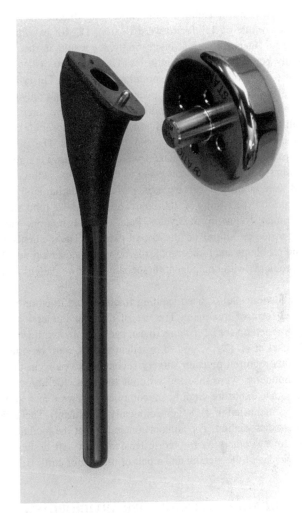

Fig. 4. Auxiliary locking pin sometimes used for taper stability, particularly in nonsymmetric head designs.

Clinical results with the modular TSA are limited both in number and duration of follow-up. Only two reports on the use of modular TSA [1,44] and one report on the use of modular hemiarthroplasty for fractures of the proximal humerus [24] were found in the literature.

Fenlin et al. [1] reported on 40 patients (mean age 62 years) who underwent TSA for a variety of shoulder pathologies. At an average follow-up of 4.5 years, the results were comparable to those reported for nonmodular systems. Pain relief was achieved in over

93% of patients and was not correlated with underlying diagnosis. Active range of motion increased an average of 35° for forward flexion, 18° for external rotation, and four vertebral levels for internal rotation. Interestingly, the results in rheumatoid arthritis patients were slightly better than in osteoarthritics. There was no evidence, however, to suggest that this was due to the use of a modular prosthesis. Thirty-five percent of patients developed glenoid radiolucent lines greater than 2 mm, but only one patient had pain necessitating removal of the glenoid component. There were three revision operations performed, all related to the glenoid component (two for loosening). There were no cases of dissociation at the modular head or glenoid components. The authors concluded that modularity helps restore soft tissue balance, which they believe is important to minimize wear and prevent component loosening due to asymmetric loading. In addition, all revision operations were facilitated by the presence of a modular humeral head.

Gartsman [44] reported the results of 100 consecutive modular total shoulder arthroplasties with a minimum follow-up of 2 years. Pain, range of motion, and activities of daily living were reported as "improved" in 95% of patients. The incidence of such complications as wound problems and radiographically observed loosening was 20%; however, there were no problems with component dissociation, and no patient underwent revision surgery.

Hemiarthroplasty for four-part or head-splitting fractures and fracture-dislocations has become an accepted form of treatment. The use of modular humeral replacement for these injuries was reported on for 22 patients (mean age 70 years) with average follow-up of 3 years by Moeckel et al. [24]. Good to excellent results were reported for 90% of patients. Two patients required revision surgery secondary to pain; in these two situations, glenoid components were inserted without the need for humeral component removal to gain adequate exposure. Significant complications were few, although heterotopic ossification was identified in 41% (none clinically significant). There were no problems with component dissociation. The authors concluded that the modular design offers several advantages, most notably more precise tensioning of soft tissues and improved exposure during revisions of the glenoid and repair of the rotator cuff.

FAILURE MODES OF MODULAR SHOULDER ARTHROPLASTY

Glenohumeral joint translation and the relative position in the sagittal plane create shear forces as compared to the compressive forces that predominate in the hip. This is of great significance with regard to wear patterns and component dissociation, which appears to occur with a higher incidence in TSA. In 1990, Driessnack et al. [36] reported the failure of three TSAs due to dissociation of the two-piece metal-backed glenoid component. In 1991, Cooper and Brems [37] described a case of recurrent disassembly of a humeral component; in their discussion, they noted that shear forces may have been a contributing factor. More recently, Sisto et al. [38] reported a similar episode of taper lock failure resulting in dissociation of a humeral component and similarly attributed it to the lack of compressive forces. It is important to note that both patients in these studies had rotator cuff deficiencies, which could create eccentric loading. In addition, any compressive force created by the rotator cuff to maintain the taper lock would be absent. Sisto et al. went on to caution that previous rotator cuff arthropathy may be a contraindication to use of a modular prosthesis due to the increased risk of dissociation. Another possible cause could be impingement of the rim of the prosthetic head on the acromion during extremes of motion.

The largest series of modular prostheses dissociations was reported by Blevins et al. [21], who reported on 12 humeral head dissociations (6 were available for inspection) and noted that the retrieved specimens had no evidence of corrosion. In addition, pull-off strengths were normal in bench testing performed after retrieval. They concluded that the primary cause of in vivo implant dissociation was improper initial seating and that as little as 0.02 mL of fluid (blood, water, or oil) contamination in the Morse-taper prior to impaction would reduce the mean dissociation force by a factor of over 10 (2966 N vs. 240 N) [21]. This risk factor also prevails in the hip, but may be overcome by the greater compressive forces. This possibility of taper failure and dissociation has led at least two authors to recommend nonmodular humeral prostheses for certain circumstances [37,38].

SUMMARY

It will be difficult to draw definitive conclusions regarding the benefits of modular TSA until long-term results become available. The two modular TSA studies discussed [1,44], however, did demonstrate results comparable to those for nonmodular designs in terms of pain relief and functional improvement. Radiolucent lines of the glenoid component continue to be a constant finding, even with modular prostheses, which is of concern in light of the conclusions of Torchia et al. [43]. Revision rates were found to be slightly lower in modular TSA patients (7.5% vs. 11% in nonmodular TSAs), but this finding cannot be considered valid until appropriate follow-up studies are performed. Isolated cases of component dissociation involving 17 patients have been reported in the literature; however, this did not occur in the two modular TSA studies. Whether this is due to the specific designs studied is not known. Only long-term studies can adequately assess the role of modularity in TSA.

REFERENCES

1. Fenlin, J. M., Ramsey, M. L., Allardyce, T. J., and Frieman, B. G., "Modular Total Shoulder Replacement," *Clinical Orthopaedics and Related Research,* Vol. 307, 1994, pp. 37–46.
2. Wirth, M. A. and Rockwood, C. A., "Complications of Shoulder Arthroplasty," *Clinical Orthopaedics,* Vol. 307, 1994, pp. 47-69.

3. Neer, C. S., "Articular Replacement for the Humeral Head," *Journal of Bone and Joint Surgery,* Vol. 37A, No. 2, 1995, pp. 215-228.
4. Coughlin, M. J., Morris, J. M., and West, W. F., "The Semiconstrained Total Shoulder Arthroplasty," *Journal of Bone and Joint Surgery,* Vol. 61A, 1979, p. 574.
5. Post, M., Haskell, S. S., and Jablon, M., "Total Shoulder Replacement with a Constrained Prosthesis," *Journal of Bone and Joint Surgery,* Vol. 62A, 1980, p. 327.
6. Post, M., Jablon, M., Miller, H., and Singh, M., "Constrained Total Shoulder Replacement: A Critical Review," *Clinical Orthopaedics and Related Research,* Vol. 144, 1979, p. 135.
7. Neer, C. S., Watson, K. C., and Stanton, F. J., "Recent Experience in Total Shoulder Replacement," *Journal of Bone and Joint Surgery,* Vol. 64A, No. 3, 1982, pp. 319-337.
8. Neer, C. S. "Replacement Arthroplasty for Glenohumeral Osteoarthritis." *Journal of Bone and Joint Surgery,* Vol. 56A, 1974, pp. 1-13.
9. Cofield, R. H., "Total Shoulder Arthroplasty with the Neer Prosthesis," *Journal of Bone and Joint Surgery,* Vol. 66A, 1984, pp. 899-906.
10. American Academy of Orthopaedic Surgeons, AAOS Bulletin, Vol. 40, 1992, p. 65.
11. Harris, W. H., "A New Total Hip Implant," *Clinical Orthopaedics and Related Research,* Vol. 81, 1971, p. 105.
12. Collier, J. P., Mayor, M. B., Jensen, R. E., Surprenant, V. A., Surprenant, H. P., McNamara, J. L., and Belec, L., "Mechanisms of Failure of Modular Prostheses," *Clinical Orthopaedics and Related Research,* Vol. 285, 1992, pp. 129-139.
13. Cook, S. D., Barrack, R. L., and Clemow, A. J. T., "Corrosion and Wear at the Modular Interfaceof Uncemented Femoral Stems," *Journal of Bone and Joint Surgery,* Vol. 76B, No. 1, 1994, pp. 68-73.
14. Lieberman, J. R., Rimnac, C. M., Garvin, K. L., Klein, R. W., and Salvati, E. A., "An Analysis of the Head-Neck Taper Interface in Retrieved Hip Prosthses," *Clinical Orthopaedics and Related Research,* Vol. 300, 1994, pp. 162-167.
15. Barrack, R. L., Burke, D. W., Cook, S. D., Skinner, H. B., and Harris, W. H., "Complications Related to Modularity of Total Hip Components," *Journal of Bone and Joint Surgery,* Vol. 75B, No. 5, 1993, pp. 688-692.
16. Cook, S. D., Barrack, R. L., Baffes, G. C., Clemow, A. J. T., Serekian, P., Dong, N., and Kester, M. A., "Wear and Corrosion of Modular Interfaces in Total Hip Replacements," *Clinical Orthopaedics and Related Research,* Vol. 298, 1994, pp. 80-88.
17. Collier, J. P., Surprenant, V. A., Jensen, R. E., Mayor, M. B., and Surprenant, H. P., "Corrosion Between the Components of Modular Femoral Hip Prostheses," *Journal of Bone and Joint Surgery,* Vol. 74B, No. 4, 1992, pp. 511-517.
18. Skinner, H. B., "Current Biomaterial Problems in Implants." In: *AAOS Instructional Course Lectures,* Vol. 41, 1992, pp. 137-144.
19. Bobyn, J. D., Tanzer, M., Krygier, J. J., Dujovne, A. R., and Brooks, C. E., "Concerns with Modularity in Total Hip Arthroplasty," *Clinical Orthopaedics and Related Research,* Vol. 298, 1994, pp. 27-36.
20. Chao, E. Y., Suh, J. K., and Grabowski, J., "Mechanical Strength and Critical Stress

Distribution of Morse Taper Lock in Modular Segmental Prosthesis Design." *Transactions of the 38th Annual Meeting of the Orthopaedic Research Society,* 1992, p. 310.

21. Blevins, F. T., Warren, R. F., Deng, X., and Torzilli, P. A., "Dissociation of Humeral Shoulder Arthroplasty Components." *Journal of Bone and Joint Surgery,* Vol. 3, No. 1, Pt. 2, 1994, p. S75.

22. McKellop, H. A., Sarmiento, A., Brien, W., and Park, S. H., "Interface Corrosion of a Modular Head Total Hip Prosthesis," *Journal of Arthroplasty,* Vol. 7, No. 3), 1992, pp. 291-294.

23. Sauer, W., Kovacs, P., Varnavas, J., and Beals, N., *Potential Corrosion-Related Phenomena at Head/Taper Interfaces,* Smith & Nephew Richards, Inc., Memphis, TN, 1993

24. Moeckel, B. H., Dines, D. M., Warren, R. F., and Altchek, D. W., "Modular Hemiarthroplasty for Fractures of the Proximal Part of the Humerus," *Journal of Bone and Joint Surgery,* Vol. 74A, No. 6, 1992, pp. 884-889.

25. Franklin, J. L., Barrett, W. P., Jackins, S. E., and Matsen, F. A., "Glenoid Loosening in Total Shoulder Arthroplasty," *Journal of Arthroplasty* Vol. 3, 1988, p. 39.

26. Hawkins, R. J., Bell, R. H., and Jallay, B., "Total Shoulder Arthroplasty," *Clinical Orthopaedics and Related Research,* Vol. 242, 1989, p. 188.

27. Dines, D. M., and Warren, R. F., "Modular Shoulder Hemiarthroplasty for Acute Fractures," *Clinical Orthopaedics and Related Research,* Vol. 307, 1994, pp. 18-26.

28. Harryman, D. T., Sidles, J. A., Harris, S. L., Lippitt, S. B., and Matsen, F. A., "The Effect of Articular Conformity and the Size of the Humeral Head Component on Laxity and Motion after Glenohumeral Arthroplasty." *Journal of Bone and Joint Surgery,* Vol. 77A, No. 4, 1995, pp. 555-563.

29. Severt, R., Thomas, B. T., Tsenter, M. J., Amstutz, H. C., and Kabo, J. M., "The Influence of Conformity and Constraint on Translational forces and Frictional Torque in Total Arthroplasty." *Clinical Orthopaedics and Related Research,* Vol. 292, 1993, pp. 151-158.

30. Vaesel, M. T. and Olsen, B. S., "Stability of the Shoulder after Hemiarthroplasty with a Modular Prosthesis," *Journal of Shoulder and Elbow Surgery,* Vol. 4, No. 1, Pt. 2, 1995, p. S27, 1995.

31. Friedman, R. J., An, Y., Chokeski, R., and Kessler, L., "Anatomic and Biomechanical Study of Glenohumeral Contact," *Journal of Shoulder and Elbow Surgery,* Vol. 3, No. 1, Pt. 2, 1994, p. S35.

32. Pagnani, M. J. and Warren, R. F., "Stabilizers of the Glenohumeral Joint," *Journal of Shoulder and Elbow Surgery,* Vol. 3, No. 3, 1994, pp. 173-187.

33. Ballmer, F. T., Lippitt, S. B., Romeo, A. A., and Matsen, F. A., "Total Shoulder Arthroplasty: Some Considerations Related to Glenoid Surface Contact," *Journal of Shoulder and Elbow Surgery,* Vol. 3, No. 5, 1994, pp. 299-306.

34. Weinstein, S. L. and Buckwalter, J. A. (Eds.), *Turek's Orthopaedics,* 5th ed., Lippincott, Philadelphia, 1994.

35. Harryman, D. T., Sidles, J. A., Clark, J. M., McQuade, K. J., Gibb, T. D., and Matsen,

F. A., "Translation of the Humeral Head on the Glenoid with Passive Glenohumeral Motion," *Journal of Bone and Joint Surgery,* Vol. 72A, 1990, pp. 1334-1343.

36. Driessnack, R. P., Ferlic, D. C., and Wiedel, J. D., "Dissociation of the Glenoid Component in Total Shoulder Arthroplasty." *Journal of Arthroplasty,* Vol. 5, 1990, pp. 15-18.

37. Cooper, R. A. and Brems, J. J., "Recurrent Disassembly of a Modular Humeral Prosthesis," *Journal of Arthroplasty,* Vol. 6, No. 4, 1991, pp. 375-377.

38. Sisto, D. J., France, M. P., Blazina, M. E., and Hirsh, L. C., "Disassembly of a Modular Humeral Prosthesis." *Journal of Arthroplasty,* Vol. 8, No. 6, 1993, pp. 653-655.

39. Friedman, R. J., Laberge, M., and Dooley, R. L., "Finite Element Modeling of the Glenoid Component: An Effect of the Design Parameters on Stress Distribution," In: *Orthopaedic Knowledge Update 4,* J. Frymoyer, Ed., American Academy of Orthopaedic Surgeons, Rosemont, IL, 1993.

40. Neer II, C. S., "Replacement Arthroplasty for Glenohumeral Arthritis." *Journal of Bone and Joint Surgery,* Vol. 56A, 1974, pp. 1-13.

41. Pollock, R. G., Higgs, G. B., Codd, T. P., Weinstein, D. M., Self, E. B., Flatow, E. L., and Bigliani, L. U., "Total Shoulder Replacement for the Treatment of Glenohumeral Arthritis," *Journal of Shoulder and Elbow Surgery,* Vol. 4, No. 1, Pt. 2, 1995, p. S12.

42. Zuckerman, J. D. and Cuomo, F., "Glenohumeral Arthroplasty: A Critical Review of Indications and Preoperative Considerations." *Bulletin of the Hospital for Joint Diseases,* Vol. 52, No. 2, 1993, pp. 21-30.

43. Torchia, M. E., Cofield, R. H., and Settergren, C. R., "Total Shoulder Arthroplasty with the Neer Prosthesis: Long-Term Results." *Journal of Shoulder and Elbow Surgery,* Vol. 4, No. 1, Pt. 2, 1995, p. S12.

44. Gartsman, G. M., "Modular Shoulder Arthroplasty," *Journal of Shoulder and Elbow Surgery,* Vol. 4, No. 1, Pt. 2, 1995, p. S56.

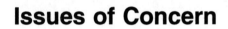

Issues of Concern

Stuart B. Goodman, [1] Phil Huie, [3] Yong Song,[4] Mike O'Connor,[5] Steven T. Woolson,[6] William J. Maloney, [7] David J. Schurman, [8] and Richard Sibley [9]

THE FIBROUS TISSUE INTERFACE SURROUNDING WELL-FIXED, REVISED, CEMENTLESS ACETABULAR COMPONENTS FOR HIP REPLACEMENT

REFERENCE: Goodman, S.B., Huie, P., Song, Y., O'Connor, M., Woolson S.T., Maloney, W.J., Schurman, D.J., and Sibley, R., "**The Fibrous Tissue Interface Surrounding Well-Fixed, Revised Cementless Acetabular Components for Hip Replacement,** *Modularity of Orthopedic Implants, ASTM STP 1301,* Donald E. Marlowe, Jack E. Parr, and Michael B. Mayor, Eds., American Society for Testing and Materials, 1997.

Abstract: Ten well-fixed, cementless, metal-backed acetabular components were revised due to recurrent hip dislocation, polyethylene wear or during femoral revision due to aseptic loosening. Eight cups were modular and two cups were nonmodular. Seven of the eight modular cups were fixed with one or more screws; the two nonmodular cups had two pegs but no screws for fixation. The cups were revised after a period of 3.5-72 months. The fibrous tissue surrounding the implant was harvested, and frozen sections were processed using immunohistochemistry and in situ hybridization. The tissue formed a thin, gritty, incomplete fibrous layer that was tightly adherent to the surface of the metal-backed components. Scattered macrophages and lymphocytes were present within the fibrous stroma in all tissues. Gross, black metallic staining of 3 tissues was associated with increased cellularity. Generally, macrophages expressed mRNA for IL-1, IL-6, PDGFa, and TNFa, and fibroblasts were TGFb positive; these factors are known to modulate the remodeling of bone. No relationship was found between the cellular and cytokine profiles and modularity, the type of metal backing, the presence of screws or the time in situ. The fibrous tissue surrounding well-fixed, cementless, metal-backed acetabular cups undergoing revision surgery contained many of the cellular elements and cytokines associated with loosening and osteolysis.

KEYWORDS: total joint replacement, cementless acetabular cups, modularity, well-fixed, immunohistochemistry, in situ hybridization

[1] Associate Professor and Chief, [3] Research Associate, [4] Research Assistant, [5] Clinical Professor, [6] Clinical Associate Professor, [7] Professor, Division of Orthopaedic Surgery and [2] Senior Research Associate, [8] Professor, Department of Pathology, Stanford University School of Medicine, 300 Pasteur Drive, Stanford, California, 94305.

Cementless implants are frequently used during total hip replacement. On the acetabular side, these devices are usually press fit and employ porous coating, and screws or pegs to supplement fixation. Cook et al. found that only a small proportion of the available pore supplement fixation. Cook et al. found that only a small proportion of the available pore space (<10%) within well-fixed, metal backed acetabular cups actually contained ingrown bone [1]. Although others have reported a more extensive amount of bone ingrowth [2,3], the biological characteristics of the remaining fibrous tissue at the cup-bone interface are generally unknown. This tissue is of critical importance for several reasons. First, further study of the properties of the interface may shed light on the processes of osseointegration of cementless implants [4]. Second, because the fibrous tissue interface may provide a conduit for the migration of particulate debris along the interface, this tissue may provide further insight into the processes of loosening and osteolysis [5-7].

In the present study we assess the properties of the fibrous tissue surrounding well-fixed, metal-backed acetabular cups undergoing revision surgery, using the techniques of histology, immunohistochemistry and in situ hybridization. The latter two methods are able to demonstrate the cellular elements and cytokine production within the interfacial tissue. We hypothesized that many of the cell types and cytokines previously associated with loosening and osteolysis would also be found in the tissues surrounding well-fixed implants undergoing revision and that these implants may represent an early form of prosthetic loosening [8,9].

MATERIALS AND METHODS

The cases included in this study are part of an ongoing prospective, consecutive series of total joint replacements undergoing surgical revision [8,9]. None of the 10 cementless metal-backed acetabular components included in this study were clinically or radiographically loose. Seven of the cups were revised due to recurrent hip dislocation, two were changed during revision of a loose, articulating femoral component, and one cup was revised due to polyethylene wear. Eight cups were modular (i.e. the parts were assembled together during surgery) and two cups were non-modular (i.e. the components of the cup were pre-assembled at the factory and could not be disassembled and exchanged at surgery). Seven of the eight modular cups were fixed with one or more screws; the two non-modular cups had two pegs but no screws for fixation. The cups were revised after a period of 3.5-49 months (modular), and 60-72 months (non-modular).

At surgery, a tissue specimen was harvested from the fibrous interface surrounding the dome of the implant and immersed in physiological saline while being transported to the laboratory. Tissue specimens approximately 5 mm in diameter were placed into BEEM capsules containing optimum cutting temperature (OCT) media (Miles, Elkhart, IN). The capsules were immediately frozen in liquid nitrogen and stored at -70°C until processed. Serial six micron sections were cut with a cryostat (Cambridge Instruments, Buffalo, NY) and mounted on microscope slides that had been pre-baked for 3 hours at 204°C.

Immunohistochemistry

Monoclonal antibodies that are specific for the surface antigens of a particular cell type were utilized in a sandwich technique [10]. Positive cells were visualized using a chromagen, diaminobenzidene, that caused the cell to appear brown. The slide was counterstained with hematoxylin, so that the background cells that had not reacted with the monoclonal antibody could be visualized. Quantitation of both the positively and negatively staining cells was then performed [10].

Technique--The mounted 6 μm thick frozen sections were fixed in absolute acetone at -20°C for one hour. The sections were incubated at room temperature, sequentially, in monoclonal mouse primary antibody, rabbit anti-mouse immunoglobulins, swine anti-rabbit immunoglobulins, and rabbit peroxidase anti-peroxidase (Dako, Carpinteria, CA). The sections were washed in phosphate buffered saline (PBS) for 20 minutes after each antibody step. Positively stained cells were visualized with diaminobenzidine, 0.01% H_2O_2, 0.3% sodium azide in 0.05 M Tris buffer pH 7.6. The slides were counterstained with Gill's hematoxylin number 3, dehydrated and mounted.

The following panel of monoclonal antibodies was used in this study to identify the presence of certain cell types, which are named according to their cluster designation (CD) and other terminology: macrophages (EMB11, CD68), total number of T lymphocytes (Leu 4, CD3 and T11), T helper lymphocytes (Leu 3A, CD4), and cytotoxic/suppressor T lymphocytes (Leu 2A, CD8) (Table 1). The diluent solution alone was used as a negative control (to account for endogenous peroxidase production). Positive controls included biopsies from cardiac and renal tissues harvested from the transplantation service. A few specimens were also processed using the mouse antihuman fibroblast antibody 5B5 that is specific for the beta subunit of prolyl-4-hydroxylase, and the Leu M3 antibody for activated macrophages.

TABLE 1- - Monoclonal antibodies used in the immunohistochemistry studies

Monoclonal Antibody	Target cell
EMB 11 (CD68)[V]	Human macrophages
Leu M3*	Activated human macrophages
Leu 4 (CD3)*	Human T cells
T11**	A pan T cell marker found in human E rosetting positive lymphocytes.
Leu 3A (CD4)*	Human T helper/inducer cells (cross reacts with monocytes/macrophages)
Leu 2A (CD8)*	Human T cytotoxic/suppressor cells
5B5[V]	ß subunit of prolyl-4-hydroxylase on fibroblasts

* Becton Dickinson, Mountain View, CA., USA

** Coulter Immunology, Hialeah, FL., USA;   V DAKO Corp., Carpinteria, CA., USA

In Situ Hybridization

Cytokines are proteins that have autocrine and paracrine functions [11, 12]. These substances typically have a very short half life, and are therefore difficult to assay in vivo. During in situ hybridization, probes of singled stranded DNA are constructed that are complementary to a target sequence on messenger RNA (mRNA) for a specific cytokine or growth factor [13, 14]. Cells that contain the mRNA for a specific cytokine are visualized using a reporter enzyme, that is indirectly attached to the specific probe-mRNA complex. When an appropriate substrate is added to the complex, a color change is seen in the cytoplasm within the cells. A counterstain is also employed, enabling the visualization of negatively staining cells.

To minimize extraneous cross-reactivity, a thorough search in GENBANK (Los Alamos, NM) was first performed to ensure that the complementary DNA (cDNA) probes used in the in situ hybridization studies did not match any housekeeping gene sequences for common cellular proteins. Probes of a uniform length (30 base pairs) and G:C ratio (0.6 - 0.7) were employed and the method of tissue processing was standardized.

   Technique--Messenger RNA sequences were obtained from GENBANK (Los Alamos, NM). Selected sequences were commercially synthesized (Operon, Alameda, CA) and biotinylated at the 3' end using biotin-11-dUTP-biotin (Sigma, St. Louis, MO), and DNA deoxynucleotidylexotransferase (Gibco, Gaithersburg, MD). Prelabeled biotinylated probes were also obtained for some sequences (Genetics Research, Huntsville, AL). After preliminary studies using a large panel of probes, the following human antisense probes were selected for detailed in situ hybridization analysis: interleukin 1 alpha (IL-1a) and beta (IL-1b), interleukin 2 (IL-2), interleukin 6 (IL-6), transforming growth factor beta (TGF-b), tumor necrosis factor alpha (TNFa), and gamma interferon (gINF). A few selected specimens were processed using probes for platelet derived growth factor alpha (PDGFa). Poly-thymidine (poly-t) was used as a positive control (poly-t binds to the poly A tail of mRNA within a cell). Negative controls included an antisense probe to Epstein Barr virus (EBV), labeled sense probes, and hybridization solution without labeled probe (Table 2).

The mounted, six micron sections were fixed for 10 minutes in 4% paraformaldehyde in physiological, phosphate buffered saline (PBS), pH 7.8, at room temperature. The slides were then washed in 3 changes of PBS/10% ethanol, dehydrated in 95% and absolute ethanol and allowed to air dry for 30 min. Working hybridization solutions were prepared with probe concentrations between 0.5 -2.0 ng/μl. The working hybridization solution was applied to tissue slices and allowed to incubate at 42°C for 1 hour. The slides were washed in 5xSSC (saline, sodium citrate) and 2xSSC. Excess 2xSSC was removed and Streptavidin-peroxidase (Dako, Carpinteria, CA) in 0.1 M Tris-Saline, pH 7.5 (1:500) was added to each section and incubated for 1 hour at room temperature. The slides were washed in 0.1 M Tris-saline, pH 7.5, 3 x 5 minutes. The color reaction was visualized with diaminobenzidine, H_2O_2. The sections were counterstained with Gill's hematoxylin number 3, dehydrated and mounted.

TABLE 2 - -**Probes examined in the in situ hybridization studies**

Cytokine/growth factor	Function
IL-1a and IL-1b	produced by many cell types including macrophages. IL-1 activates macrophages, neutrophils and endothelial cells, stimulates fibroblasts and osteoclasts, and induces prostaglandin E2 and collagenase synthesis. IL-1a and b are producers of two distinct genes; the two proteins have 25% homology and recognize the same cell surface receptors.
IL-2	produced by T helper cells; IL-2 stimulates growth and proliferation of T and B cells and activated killer T lymphocytes.
IL-6	produced by macrophages, T cells, fibroblasts and other cell types; IL-6 activates T and B cells, induces B cells to differentiate and secrete immunoglobulins.
TGFb	produced by T cells, activated macrophages, and other cell types; TGFb stimulates fibroblast growth, extracellular matrix formation, suppresses T and B cell proliferation. TGFb also stimulates osteoblasts and inhibits osteoclasts.
TNFa	produced by activated lymphocytes, monocytes, macrophages and other cells; TNFa stimulates fibroblasts and granulocytes; many of the effects are similar to IL-1.
gIFN	produced by T cells; gIFN has antiviral activity and enhances activated killer cells.
PDGFa	produced by macrophages, platelets, endothelial cells and osteoclasts to resorb bone, induces collagenase and prostaglandin production, and is chemotactic for fibroblasts, monocytes and neutrophils.
Poly T	a probe binding to the poly A tail of mRNA (a positive control)

Assessment

Hematoxylin and eosin stained sections were first examined to discern the general histomorphological features of the tissue. A quantitative assessment was performed for each stain/probe by calculating the percentage of positively staining cells using a light microscope and grid counting technique. Fifty to seventy-five cells were classified in each of the four quadrants of the tissue section, yielding a minimum of 200 cell counts per stain/probe. The first quadrant for cell counting was chosen randomly on the slide and labelled the "12 o'clock" position; the second, third and fourth quadrants for counting were then automatically designated, according to the 3, 6 and 9 o'clock positions. The data was tabulated and entered into a MacIntosh Centris computer using Statview (Abacus Concepts, Berkeley, CA, USA).

RESULTS

Gross Examination

All of the revised cups were extracted with great difficulty, even after any screws were removed. The surface of the metal backing was covered with variable amounts of soft tissue and cancellous bone; the bone was mainly located at the acetabular dome and around the screw holes. When the cancellous bone apposed to the cup was removed with a rongeur, a fibrous, smooth, soft tissue interface was frequently found interposed between the cup and the bone. The soft tissue formed a thin, gritty, fibrous, whitish-tan layer that was tightly adherent to the surface of the metal-backed components or the underlying bone. Three of the cups were associated with gross black staining of the surrounding tissues (cases 3,4 and 7).

Histology, histochemistry and in situ hybridization (Table 3 and Figure 1)

The fibrous tissue harvested from the immediate bone-implant interface was generally hypocellular. Fibrocartilage was occasionally noted. Scattered macrophages and lymphocytes were present within the fibrous stroma in all tissues, as early as 3 months postoperatively. The macrophages frequently expressed the mRNA for IL-1, Il-6, PDGFa and TNFa; fibroblasts often expressed TGFb mRNA. There was no relationship between the cellular and cytokine profiles and the type of metal backing (titanium or cobalt chrome alloy), modularity, the presence of screws or the time in situ. In general, particulate debris (polyethylene or metallic) was occasionally located within scattered macrophages, but this was not a conspicuous histologic feature, compared to tissues from loose implants with/without osteolysis [8,9]. However, metallic and polyethylene particles within sheets of macrophages were found in the tissues from the three implants associated with gross black staining. These tissues generally contained the greatest absolute numbers of all cell types, and some of the greatest proportions of cells expressing the mRNA for IL-1b, IL-6, PDGFa and TGFb (Table 3).

DISCUSSION

The success of cementless acetabular components for total joint replacement is well established [2,3]. Although complete osseointegration of metal-backed acetabular implants has not been achieved, the clinical results using this method of stabilization have been most impressive [1,2,3]. Retrieved tissues from autopsy cases and from well-fixed revised components can provide valuable information concerning the processes of

TABLE 3- - Demographic data including the percentage of positive cells for each monoclonal antibody and cytokine tested

	Age	Original Diagnosis	Reason for Revision	Prev OR	In Situ	Shell Material
1	57	ON	recurrent dislocation	1	4 mo	Ti
2	71	ON	recurrent dislocation	1	7 mo	Ti
3	57	OA	recurrent dislocation	2	20 mo	Ti
4	23	OS	polyethylene wear	1	24 mo	Ti
5	76	OA	recurrent dislocation	3	24 mo	CoCr
6	76	OA	femoral revision	2	32 mo	Ti
7	52	OA	femoral revision	3	39 mo	Ti
8	56	Trauma	recurrent dislocation	2	48 mo	CoCr
9	59	OA	recurrent dislocation	1	49 mo	CoCr
10	62	Trauma	recurrent dislocation	2	72 mo	CoCr

	Emb 11	leu 2A	leu 3A	leu 4	T11	leu M3	5B5
1	41	11	15	17	25	33	39
2	62	17	8	11	29	17	5
3	38	17	28	19	40	33	68
4	78	19	58	42	54	61	22
5	43	10	21	11	7	31	NA
6	48	22	35	25	26	NA	NA
7	97	12	9	38	34	88	19
8	14	29	39	18	13	NA	NA
9	88	12	14	25	30	57	9
10	85	20	59	34	29	52	17

	Diluent	IL-1a	IL-1b	IL-2	IL-6	TGFb	TNFa
1	0	23	20	1	87	37	15
2	0	5	16	1	40	34	9
3	0	9	38	1	91	75	36
4	2	72	56	63	74	57	77
5	3	32	31	NA	40	0	47
6	0	NA	NA	NA	NA	0	NA
7	0	90	77	0	98	87	67
8	0	36	56	33	50	0	59
9	0	19	20	1	71	38	10
10	1	15	32	30	60	67	27

TABLE 3- - Demographic data including the percentage of positive cells for each monoclonal antibody and cytokine tested (continued)

	PDGFa	gIFN	Poly t	Hybridization Solution
1	23	0	65	0
2	22	1	30	0
3	74	1	63	0
4	66	79	73	0
5	NA	31	28	0
6	NA	NA	NA	NA
7	93	6	83	0
8	NA	53	60	0
9	39	0	29	0
10	63	29	63	0

LEGEND

OA = osteoarthritis
ON = osteonecrosis
Trauma = traumatic arthritis
Femoral revision = cup revised with loose femoral component
Prev OR = number of previous operations on that hip
In Situ = time prosthesis was in situ
Shell Material = material composition of the acetabular shell
Ti = TI 6-Al 4-V alloy
CoCr = cobalt chrome alloy
NA = not available

Abbreviations for the different cell antigens and cytokines can be found in Tables 1 and 2.

FIG. 1- - Immunohistochemistry and in situ hybridization of the retrieved tissue from a revised cementless acetabular cup

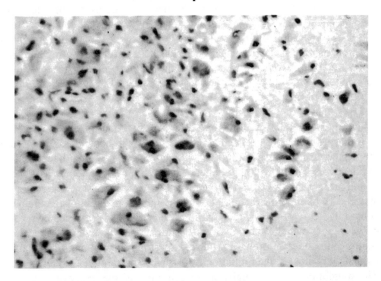

C) In situ hybridization using a probe for interleukin 1 beta. The cell nuclei stain intensely. Positive cells for interleukin 1 beta have a greyish cytoplasmic staining. magnification = 400X

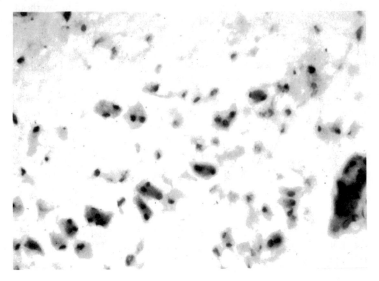

D) In situ hybridization using a probe for interleukin 6. The cell nuclei stain intensely. Positive cells for interleukin 6 have a greyish cytoplasmic staining. magnification = 400X

osseointegration of cementless implants. The fibrous tissue examined in this study was from well-fixed acetabular components that were revised due to recurrent dislocation, polyethylene wear, or during femoral revision due to aseptic loosening. It is probable that our study represents, in a qualitative way, failure of the implant and an early stage of loosening. Thus, the findings in this study are not analagous to the situation in which a well-fixed, problem-free acetabular component has been harvested during autopsy [2,3]. Furthermore, our studies require fresh tissue that is immediately frozen, to prevent posthumous autolytic degradation of the retrieved tissue. For this reason, the present study can not be performed using autopsy retrieved specimens.

Both the quantity and cellularity of the harvested soft tissue in this study was much less compared to tissues from loose cemented or cementless components [8,9]. Despite this, the fibrous tissue stroma surrounding well-fixed, cementless metal-backed acetabular cups contained many of the cellular elements and cytokines previously associated with loosening and osteolysis [8,9,12,15-19]. In this study, no relationship was found between the cellular and cytokine profiles and the time in situ, the material of the metal backing (titanium or cobalt chrome alloy), modularity of the cup or the presence of screws. The three cups with gross metallic staining of the tissues all had an obvious source of metallic debris from metal on metal fretting. In these tissues, the surrounding fibrous tissue may have provided a conduit for the migration of particles and foreign body cells around the cup.   The membrane was generally more cellular and the expression of cytokines commonly associated with adverse bone remodeling was more conspicuous in these 3 cases [8,9].

Modular acetabular cups enable surgeons to revise the polyethylene liner without revising the metallic shell. This might be useful when revising a femoral component containing a different sized femoral head, in cases associated with polyethylene wear (especially in younger patients), and when exchanging a standard liner for one with enhanced stability. The number of well-fixed, metal-backed acetabular cups in this series is small. Despite this, our study has shown that well-fixed modular cups that are assembled at surgery will not lead to a less desirable interface tissue than if the cups were were pre-assembled by the manufacturer, and could not be disassembled and revised at surgery.

Acknowledgement: This study was supported in part by a grant from Howmedica.

REFERENCES

1. Cook, S. D., "Clinical, radiographic and histologic evaluation of retrieved human noncemented porous coated implants,". J. Long-term Effects of Medical Implants. Vol. 1, No. 1, 1991, pp 11-51.

2. Pinhorz, L. E., Urban, R. M., Jacobs, J. J., Sumner, D. R., and Galante, J. O., "A qualitative study of bone and soft tissues in cementless porous-coated acetabular components retrieved at autopsy," J. Arthroplasty Vol. 8 No. 2, 1993, pp 213-225.

3. Engh, C.A., Zettl-Schaffer, K. F., Kukita, Y., Sweet, D., Jasty, M., Bragdon, C. E., "Histological and radiographic assessment of well-functioning porous-coated acetabular components. A human post-mortem retrieval study," J. Bone Jt Surg. Vol. 75-A, 1993, pp 814-823.

4. Albrektsson, T. and Albrektsson B., "Osseointegration of bone implants. A review of an alternative mode of fixation," Acta Orthop. Scand. Vol 58, 1987, pp567-577.

5. Maloney, W. J., Jasty, M., Harris, W. H., Galante, J. O., Callaghan, J. J., "Endosteal erosion in association with stable uncemented femoral components," J Bone Jt Surg. Vol. 72-A, 1990, pp 1026-34.

6. Maloney, W. J., Peters, P., Engh, C. A., and Chandler, H., "Severe osteolysis of the pelvis in association with acetabular replacement without cement," J. Bone Jt. Surg. Vol. 75-A, 1993, pp 1627-1635.

7. Schmalzried, T. P., Guttmann, D., Grecula, M., and Amstutz, H. C., "The relationship between design, position, and articular wear of acetabular components inserted without cement and the development of pelvic osteolysis," J Bone Jt Surg Vol. 76-A, 1994, pp 677-688.

8 Goodman, S. B., Sibley, R., Huie, P., Lee, K., Doshi, A., Rushdieh, B., Woolson, S. T., Maloney, W. J. and Schurman, D. J., "Loosening and osteolysis of cemented joint arthroplasties: A biological spectrum," Transactions of the Orthopaedic Research Society Vol. 19, 1994, p 839.

9 Goodman, S. B., Huie, P. and Song, Y., "Cellular profile and cytokine production in tissues surrounding revised cementless prostheses," Transactions of the Orthopaedic Research Society Vol. 20, 1995, p 744.

10. Goodman, S. B., Knoblich, G., O'Connor, M., Song, Y., Huie, P., and Sibley R. "The heterogeneity in cellular and cytokine profiles from multiple samples of tissue surrounding revised hip prostheses, " Accepted for publication, J. Biomed. Mat. Res.

11. Goldring, M. B., Goldring, S. R., "Skeletal tissue response to cytokines". Clin. Orthop. Vol. 258, 1990, pp 245-278.

12. Jiranek, W. A., Machado, M., Jasty, M., Jevsevar, D., Wolfe, H. J., Goldring, S. R., Goldberg, M. J., and Harris, W. H., "Production of cytokines around loosened cemented acetabular components. Analysis with immunohistochemical techniques and in situ hybridization," J Bone Joint Surg. Vol. 75-A, 1993, pp 863-879.

13. Myerson, D. "In situ hybridization". In: Diagnostic Immunopathology. Bhan R T and McCluskey R T (eds) Raven Press, New York. 1988; pp 475-498.

14. Nakamura, R. M. "Overview and principles of in-situ hybridization". Clinical Biochemistry Vol. 23, 1990, pp 255-259.

15. Chiba, J., Rubash, H. E., Kim, K. J., and Iwaki, Y. "The characterization of cytokines in the interace tissue from failed cementless total hip replacements with and without femoral osteolysis," Clin. Orthop. Vol. 300, 1994, pp 304-312.

16. Kim, K.J., Chiba, J., and Rubash, H. E., "In vivo and in vitro analysis of membranes from hip prostheses inserted without cement," J. Bone Jt. Surg. Vol. 76-A, 1994, pp 172-180.

17. Ohlin, A., Johnell, O., Lerner U. H., "The pathogenesis of loosening of total hip arthroplasties. The production of factors by periprosthetic tissues that stimulate in vitro bone resorption," Clin Orthop Vol. 253, 1990, pp 287-296.

18. Santavirta, S., Konttinen, Y. T., Begroth, V., Eskola, A., Tallroth, K., and Lindholm, S. "Aggressive granulomatous lesions associated with hip arthroplasty. Immunopathological studies," J. Bone Jt. Surg. Vol. 72-A, 1990, pp 252-258.

19. Santavirta, S., Kontinnen, Y.T., Hoikka, V., Eskola, A. "Immunopathological response to loose cementless acetabular components," J. Bone Jt Surg. Vol. 73-B, 1991, pp 38-42.

Robert M. Urban,[1] Joshua J. Jacobs,[1] Jeremy L. Gilbert,[2] Stephen B. Rice,[3] Murali Jasty,[4] Charles R. Bragdon,[4] and Jorge O. Galante[1]

CHARACTERIZATION OF SOLID PRODUCTS OF CORROSION GENERATED BY MODULAR-HEAD FEMORAL STEMS OF DIFFERENT DESIGNS AND MATERIALS

REFERENCE: Urban, R.M., Jacobs, J.J., Gilbert, J.L., Rice, S.B., Jasty, M., Bragdon, C.R., and Galante, J.O., **"Characterization of Solid Products of Corrosion Generated by Modular-Head Femoral Stems of Different Designs and Materials,"** *Modularity of Orthopedic Implants, ASTM STP 1301,* Donald E. Marlowe, Jack E. Parr, and Michael B. Mayor, Eds., American Society for Testing and Materials, 1997.

ABSTRACT: This paper reviews the microanalytic and histopathologic findings from studies reported previously by our laboratory describing the nature and significance of solid products of corrosion generated at modular junctions of femoral components for hip replacement. A total of twenty-five retrieved, corroded modular junctions with surrounding tissues were examined from a variety of component designs and material combinations, including head/neck couples of CoCr/CoCr, CoCr/Ti6Al4V, and Al_2O_3/CoCr. The products were examined using electron microprobe with energy-dispersive x-ray analysis, x-ray diffraction, and Fourier-transform infrared spectroscopy.

The products of corrosion identified at the modular junctions of all of the various prostheses examined were similar regardless of the implant design or materials coupled, even when a ceramic head was employed. The most prevalent corrosion product was characterized as an amorphous chromium orthophosphate hydrate-rich material. Particles of this material were identified throughout the periprosthetic tissues of most of the cases studied and at the polyethylene bearing surface of several cases. The multitude of particles generated by fragmentation of the corrosion products and the finding that they migrate to sites distant from their origin are of concern because of their potential to

---

[1] Research Associate and Administrator, Research Programs; Associate Professor and Director, Section of Biomaterials Research; and Professor and Director of the Rush Arthritis and Orthopedics Institute, respectively, Rush-Presbyterian-St. Luke's Medical Center, 1653 W. Congress Parkway, Chicago, IL 60612.

[2] Associate Professor, Division of Biological Materials and Department of Biomedical Engineering, Northwestern University, Chicago, IL 60611.

[3] Senior Electron Microscopist, McCrone Associates, Inc.; Westmont, IL 60559.

[4] Clinical Associate Professor, and Senior Research Associate, respectively, Massachusetts General Hospital and Harvard Medical School, Boston, MA 02114.

increase the production of polyethylene wear debris by a three-body wear mechanism and their direct participation in particle-induced, macrophage-mediated osteolysis.

KEYWORDS: Corrosion, hip replacement, particulate debris, biocompatibility, wear

---

One of the potential degradation products of femoral components for hip replacement that have a modular head is the solid products of corrosion that can be generated at the tapered connection. The deposition of these products at the head/neck junction was noted in many of the initial published reports on corrosion of these devices [1,2,3]. In cases of severe corrosion, the presence of these deposits is grossly apparent even to the operating surgeon at the time of revision. However, the nature of solid corrosion products and their significance to the long-term durability of joint replacements has, for the most part, remained unknown. This paper summarizes previously published efforts by our laboratory to characterize the composition of solid products of corrosion from the head/neck junctions of a variety of femoral component designs and material couples, and to determine their distribution in the periprosthetic tissues [4,5,6,7] .

MATERIALS AND METHODS

Solid corrosion products from the head/neck junction of 25 hip replacement femoral components of 10 designs from 6 manufactures were studied (Table 1). The components were selected from a collection of corroded devices that had been sent to the authors by many other surgeons. The particular cases were chosen to represent a range of designs that exhibited macroscopic corrosion, had been implanted without the use of auxiliary plates, screws, wires, or cables, and for which adequate specimens of the periprosthetic tissues were available for analyses. The prostheses had been implanted in 16 males and 9 females at a mean age of 53 years (range 26 to 68 years), and were retrieved after a mean time *in situ* of 65 months (range 8 to 99 months). The devices were removed at revision surgery in 19 cases and at autopsy in 6 cases. The reason for revision was femoral osteolysis without loosening in 8 cases, femoral osteolysis with loosening in 4 cases, femoral component aseptic loosening in 2 cases, and in 1 case each: fracture of the acetabular liner, corrosion fatigue fracture of the neck of the femoral stem, recurrent dislocation, sepsis, and acetabular osteolysis without loosening (case 22).

Twenty-four of the prostheses had cobalt-base alloy (CoCr) heads. They were coupled with cementless, porous coated titanium-6%-aluminum-4%vanadium alloy (Ti6Al4V) stems in 16 cases, cementless porous coated CoCr stems in 3 cases (cases 1, 6, and 7), and cemented CoCr stems without porous coating in 5 cases. The remaining prosthesis had an alumina (Al_2O_3) head and a CoCr stem with no porous coating and had been implanted without the use of acrylic cement. Polyethylene liners from the acetabular components of 14 of the cases were available for study. The corrosion products were isolated from the head/neck junction and the polyethylene bearing surface

TABLE 1--Retrieved implants

Case	Prosthesis Type[1]	Materials (Head/Neck)	Duration (Mos.)	Reason for Removal
1	PCA	CoCr/CoCr	24	Sepsis
2	Precoat	CoCr/CoCr	50	Autopsy
3	Precoat	CoCr/CoCr	57	Autopsy
4	Precision	CoCr/CoCr	60	Osteolysis with loosening
5	Precoat CDH	CoCr/CoCr	68	Osteolysis with loosening
6	AML	CoCr/CoCr	72	Fractured acetabular liner
7	PCA	CoCr/CoCr	85	Fracture at the neck
8	Precoat	CoCr/CoCr	96	Osteolysis with loosening
9	Autophor	Al_2O_3/CoCr	99	Aseptic loosening
10	Harris-Galante	CoCr/Ti6Al4V	8	Autopsy
11	Omniflex	CoCr/Ti6Al4V	44	Recurrent dislocation
12	Harris-Galante	CoCr/Ti6Al4V	49	Osteolysis with loosening
13	BIAS	CoCr/Ti6Al4V	54	Autopsy
14	Anatomic	CoCr/Ti6Al4V	55	Osteolysis w/o loosening
15	Taperloc	CoCr/Ti6Al4V	59	Autopsy
16	Harris-Galante	CoCr/Ti6Al4V	60	Osteolysis w/o loosening
17	Harris-Galante	CoCr/Ti6Al4V	61	Autopsy
18	Harris-Galante	CoCr/Ti6Al4V	65	Osteolysis w/o loosening
19	Harris-Galante	CoCr/Ti6Al4V	68	Aseptic loosening
20	Harris-Galante	CoCr/Ti6Al4V	70	Osteolysis w/o loosening
21	BIAS	CoCr/Ti6Al4V	72	Osteolysis w/o loosening
22	Harris-Galante	CoCr/Ti6Al4V	86	Osteolysis w/o loosening
23	Harris-Galante	CoCr/Ti6Al4V	89	Osteolysis w/o loosening
24	Harris-Galante	CoCr/Ti6Al4V	89	Osteolysis w/o loosening
25	Harris-Galante	CoCr/Ti6Al4V	97	Osteolysis with loosening

[1] PCA and Precision (Howmedica, Rutherford, NJ); Anatomic, Precoat, BIAS, and Harris-Galante (Zimmer, Warsaw, IN); AML (Depuy, Warsaw, IN); Autophor (Smith & Nephew Richards (Memphis, TN); Omniflex (Osteonics, Allendale, NJ); Taperloc (Biomet, Warsaw, IN).

and mounted on beryllium or carbon plates as previously described [4]. Samples from every case were examined by electron microprobe with energy dispersive x-ray analysis, and by x-ray diffraction using the Debye-Scherrer powder camera method. In 15 cases, the corrosion products were also characterized by Fourier-transform infrared spectroscopy (FTIR). In case 22, submicron particles of the corrosion products were prepared for examination by parallel electron energy loss spectroscopy (PEELS). PEELS was used to determine the chromium valence of corrosion products by comparison with reference samples of chromium oxide (Cr_2O_3, valence 3+), and potassium chromate (K_2CrO_4, valence 6+). Stained histologic sections of the hip joint pseudocapsule, bone-implant interface membranes, and osteolytic lesions were examined by light microscopy for the presence of particles of the corrosion products. The composition of intracellular particles was studied in unstained sections of the periprosthetic tissues using backscattered-electron scanning electron microscopy and electron microprobe analysis.

RESULTS

At the modular connection, solid corrosion products were found at two locations. They were present within the crevice formed by the bore of the head and the tapered neck, and they were deposited at the opening of the crevice around the rim of the bore and on the neck of the prosthesis just distal to the head-neck junction (Fig. 1). The nature of the corrosion products differed at these two locations.

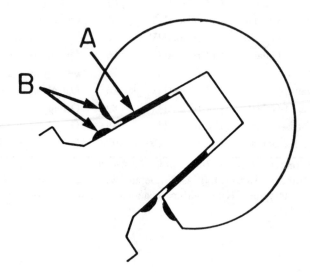

FIG. 1--Schematic drawing of the locations of the corrosion products, (A) as a thin interfacial layer within the crevice formed by the junction of the head and neck, and (B) as thicker deposits around the opening of the crevice.

Areas where the head and neck of the prostheses had been mated (A of Fig. 1) had a thin, friable interfacial layer of corrosion products covering pitted and etched surfaces of corroded metal. These deposits were black and occasionally green or violet, and 10 to 200 micrometers thick. Electron microprobe analysis indicated that the interfacial layer was composed of mixed oxides and chlorides of chromium, molybdenum, and in some of the CoCr/Ti6Al4V couples, titanium (Figure 2). The material of the interfacial layer was highly crystalline by x-ray diffraction with principal lines at 1.68, 2.19, and 2.48 angstroms. The implants from cases 6 and 7 demonstrated similar corrosion products associated with severe intergranular corrosion of the neck of CoCr porous coated femoral stems. The other 6 cases with corroded CoCr/CoCr couples did not show evidence of intergranular corrosion. In implant 5, which had an Al_2O_3 head, corrosion was limited to the neck side of the junction which was made of CoCr, but the black and green corrosion products were adherent to the inside of the ceramic head as well.

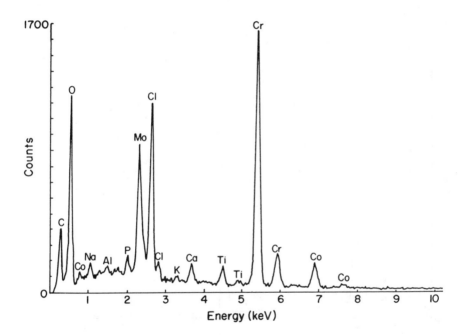

FIG. 2--Energy dispersive x-ray spectrum of the interfacial layer of corrosion products adherent to the inside of the CoCr-alloy head from Case 15. The black corrosion deposit was composed of highly crystalline, mixed oxides and chlorides of chromium and molybdenum. The specimen consisted by weight of approximately 45% oxygen, 25% chromium, 10% chlorine, 9% molybdenum, 4% cobalt, and 1% titanium with the balance consisting of sodium, sulfur, phosphorous, calcium, and aluminum.

The corrosion product around the opening of the crevice (B of Fig. 1) was identified as an amorphous chromium orthophosphate hydrate-rich material. The deposits were dark green and glassy in appearance. They were one to three millimeters in thickness and were present on the rim of the head and around the neck of the stem just distal to the head/neck junction where no corrosion of the metal was evident. Electron microprobe analysis indicated that in all of the implants this corrosion product consisted primarily of chromium, phosphorous, and oxygen (Fig. 3). Variable concentrations of calcium, molybdenum, titanium, or cobalt were often present. Low levels of other elements were also detected including aluminum, iron, potassium, sodium, sulfur, and chlorine. Comparison of the PEELS spectra collected from the chromium phosphate corrosion product from case 22 with spectra from the Cr_2O_3 (Cr valence 3+) and K_2CrO_4 (Cr valence 6+) standards indicated that the chromium valence of the corrosion product was 3+. X-ray diffraction studies of the chromium phosphate corrosion products at the opening of the crevice demonstrated that they were essentially amorphous, in contrast to the highly crystalline deposits of the interfacial layer within the crevice.

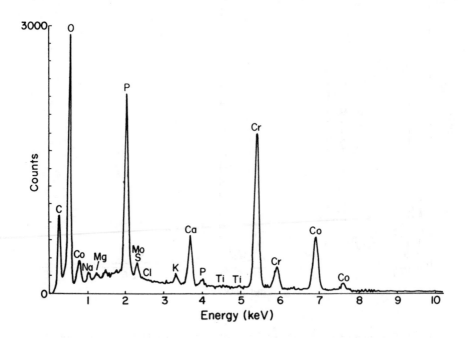

FIG. 3--Case 15. Energy-dispersive x-ray spectrum of a typical chromium phosphate corrosion product isolated from the rim of the bore in the head of a CoCr/Ti6Al4V couple. This glassy, green deposit was high in chromium, phosphorous, and oxygen. Variable concentrations of calcium, molybdenum, cobalt, and titanium were also present.

At the polyethylene bearing surface, numerous green particles, 4 to 200 micrometers in size, of the chromium phosphate corrosion product were identified by electron microprobe analyses in cases 3, 7, and 25.

FTIR spectra of the corrosion deposits at the opening of the crevice were similar for all of the fifteen implants examined by this technique and indicated that the material was a hydrated orthophosphate. The spectra were characterized by absorption bands due to water molecules between 3200 and 3400 cm^{-1} and a prominent band of phosphate absorption between 1020 and 1060 cm^{-1}. These spectra closely matched those of a reference material, chromium phosphate tetrahydrate, $CrPO_4 \cdot 4H_2O$ (Fig. 4). Spectra of the chromium phosphate corrosion products were similar from the head/neck junction, the polyethylene bearing surface, and the periprosthetic tissues (Fig. 4).

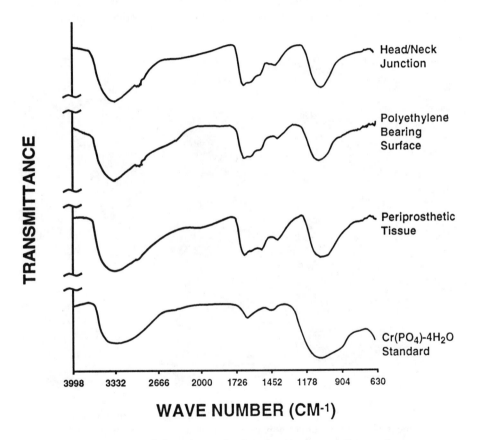

FIG. 4--FTIR spectra of chromium orthophosphate hydrate-rich corrosion products from the head/neck junction (case 16), the polyethylene bearing surface (case 7), and the joint pseudocapsule (case 3) compared to a $CrPO_4 \cdot 4H_2O$ standard.

Examination of the tissue sections revealed pale green particles of the chromium orthophosphate hydrate-rich corrosion product in the periprosthetic tissues of 23 of the 25 cases. The particles ranged in size from submicron to up to several hundred micrometers. Most of the particles were present within histiocytes, intermixed with fine polyethylene debris. The larger fragments were surrounded by foreign-body giant cells (Fig. 5). Particles of the corrosion product were not birefringent and did not stain by standard hematoxylin and eosin technique. Particles that were less than a few micrometers in size were translucent and colorless. These were more readily demonstrated by backscattered-electron SEM images in which they appeared as bright particles due to their relatively higher average atomic number. Particles of the chromium orthophosphate hydrate-rich corrosion product were detected in the joint pseudocapsule, femoral bone-implant interface membranes, and in the femoral and acetabular osteolytic lesions in all of these cases. In contrast, particles of the mixed oxides and chlorides from within the crevice formed by the mated head and neck were rarely detected in the periprosthetic tissues.

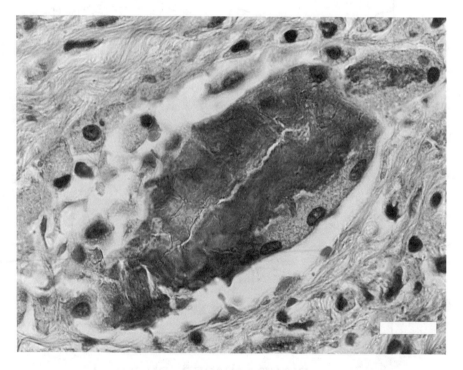

FIG. 5--Case 15. An approximately 100 micrometer, green, non-birefringent fragment of the chromium orthophosphate hydrate-rich corrosion product is surrounded by histiocytes and a flattened foreign-body giant cell in the hip joint pseudocapsule adjacent to a corroded CoCr/Ti6Al4V modular junction. (H&E; original magnification, X940; length of the bar, 20 μm).

DISCUSSION

Cobalt-chromium-molybdenum alloys are generally considered to have excellent *in vivo* corrosion resistance. However, the modular design of contemporary femoral components for hip replacement can introduce conditions which foster accelerated corrosion of these alloys [2]. The products of corrosion identified at the modular junctions of all of the various prostheses examined were similar regardless of the implant design or the materials coupled, even when a ceramic head was employed. Two distinct varieties of corrosion products were found. One was a highly crystalline interfacial layer of mixed oxides and chlorides intimately associated with the site of corrosion within the crevice formed by the mated head and neck. The other was an amorphous chromium orthophosphate hydrate-rich material deposited just outside of the crevice, apparently as a precipitate of chromium with phosphorous from the fluids of the joint cavity. These corrosion products are of concern regarding their potential local and systemic effects.

Particles of the mixed oxides and chlorides from within the crevice were found only rarely in the surrounding tissues, but abundant, fine particulate debris of the chromium phosphate corrosion product was observed in the periprosthetic tissues of most of the specimens examined. This was consistent with the more extensive deposition of this material around the opening of the crevice and its ready access to the joint cavity. These studies have also documented the migration of particulate chromium phosphate corrosion products from the modular junction to sites remote from their origin [4]. These sites include the polyethylene bearing surface, the bone-implant interface membranes, and osteolytic lesions adjacent to the distal aspect of the stem of the femoral component. Necrosis, lymphadenopathy, hypersensitivity reaction and pseudotumor formation have also been reported in association with similar corrosion products [3,8,9] .

In vitro studies of the cellular response to particles fabricated from commercial preparations of chromium phosphate indicate that the material has the capacity to stimulate bone-resorbing cytokine release from macrophages and to stimulate bone resorption in organ culture in a dose dependent manner [10]. In the present investigation, electron energy loss studies suggested a chromium valence of 3+ rather than 6+ for the corrosion product. Some authors believe that the hexavalent compounds are the more toxic form of chromium [11]. The corrosion product isolated in the present study also contained variable amounts of other metals, including, in some of the particles, substantial amounts of cobalt. Currently, very little is known regarding the chemical states and combining species of these other metals or the effects of their potential intracellular release [12].

Systemic dissemination of both soluble and particulate corrosion products from modular junctions has also been described, including the finding of chromium phosphate particles in the para-aortic lymph nodes of a patient with a corroded but otherwise successful total hip prosthesis [6,7,13]. The extent to which particulate debris migrates from joint replacement prostheses to distant organs has only recently become recognized, and presently the potential metabolic, immunologic, and oncogenic toxicity of disseminated particulate debris remains undefined [13].

The identification of chromium phosphate corrosion products at the polyethylene bearing surface indicates that these particles have the potential to accelerate the wear process through a three-body mechanism. In this manner, these corrosion products may indirectly contribute to component loosening and periprosthetic osteolysis due to the production of a greater volume of polyethylene wear debris.

The studies reviewed in this paper demonstrated the formation of similar solid products of corrosion with implants of a number of different designs and manufactures. The phenomenon appears to be generic to intraoperatively assembled femoral hip replacement prostheses with a head/neck modular connection in which at least one of the components is fabricated from CoCr-alloy [2,7]. Several large retrieval studies have reported an incidence of corrosion at head/neck junctions ranging from 9% to 23% for CoCr/CoCr couples and 35% to 37% for CoCr/Ti6Al4V couples [4,14,15]. The fact that macroscopic corrosion was not observed in the majority of specimens from those studies suggests that the problem could be avoided. Given the important advantages of the flexibility afforded the surgeon and the ability to select the head and stem materials independently, it is likely that the current widespread use of modular head prostheses will continue. Improvements in fretting corrosion resistance, however, will be necessary to ensure the durability and safety of these devices.

ACKNOWLEDGMENT

The authors gratefully acknowledge the assistance of Drs. John Gavrilovic, Wayne Paprosky, Aaron Rosenberg, John Roth, and Mitchell Sheinkop. This work was supported by grant AR39310 from the National Institute of Arthritis and Musculoskeletal and·Skin Diseases, and by Zimmer, Warsaw, IN.

REFERENCES

[1]   Collier, J.P., Suprenant, V.A., Jensen, R.E., and Mayor, M.B., "Corrosion at the Interface of Cobalt-Alloy Heads on Titanium-Alloy Stems," *Clinical Orthopaedics and Related Research,* Number 271, October 1991, pp 305-312.

[2]   Gilbert, J.L., Buckley, C.A., Jacobs, J.J., "*In vivo* Corrosion of Modular Hip Prosthesis Components in Mixed and Similar Metal Combinations. The Effect of Crevice, Stress, Motion, and Alloy Coupling," *Journal of Biomedical Materials Research,* Vol. 27, December 1993, pp 1533-1544.

[3]   Mathiesen, E.B., Lindgren, J.U., Blomgren, G.G.A., and Reinholt, F.P., "Corrosion of Modular Hip Prostheses," *The Journal of Bone and Joint Surgery,* Vol. 73-B, No. 4, July 1991, pp 569-575.

[4]   Urban, R.M., Jacobs J.J., Gilbert, J.L., and Galante, J.O., "Migration of Corrosion Products from Modular Hip Prostheses. Particle Microanalysis and Histopathological Findings," *The Journal of Bone and Joint Surgery,* Vol. 76-A, No. 9, September 1994, pp 1345-1359.

[5]   Urban, R.M., Jacobs, J.J., Tomlinson, M.J., Gavrilovic, J., and Andersen, M.E., "Migration of Corrosion Products from the Modular Head Junction to the Polyethylene Bearing Surface and Interface Membranes of Hip Prostheses," *Total Hip Revision Surgery,* Jorge O. Galante, Aaron G. Rosenberg, and John J. Callaghan, Eds., Raven Press, New York, 1995, pp 61-71.

[6]   Jacobs, J.J., Gilbert, J.L., and Urban, R.M., "Corrosion of Metallic Implants," *Advances in Operative Orthopaedics, Volume 2,* Richard N. Stauffer, Ed., Mosby, St. Louis, 1994, pp 279-319.

[7]   Jacobs, J.J., Urban, R.M., Gilbert, J.L., Skipor, A.K., Black, J., Jasty, M., and Galante, J.O., "Local and Distant Products from Modularity," *Clinical Orthopaedics and Related Research,* Number 319, October 1995, pp 94-105.

[8]   Jacobs, J.J., Urban, R.M., Wall, J., Black, J., Reid, J.D., and Veneman, L., "Unusual Foreign-Body Reaction to a Failed Total Knee Replacement: Simulation of a Sarcoma Clinically and a Sarcoid Histologically," *The Journal of Bone and Joint Surgery,* Vol. 77-A, No. 3, March 1995, pp 444-451.

[9]   Winter, G.D., "Wear and Corrosion Products in Tissues and the Reactions They Provoke," *Biocompatibility of Implant Materials,* David F. Williams, Ed., Sector, London, 1976, pp 28-39.

[10]   Jacobs, J.J., Urban, R.M., Otternes, I., Ragasa, D., Glant, T.T., "Biological Activity of Particulate Chromium-Phosphate Corrosion Products," *Transactions Society for Biomaterials,* Vol. XVIII, March 1995, p 398.

[11]   Langard, S., Norseth, T., "Chromium," *Handbook of the Toxicology of Metals, Volume 2, Specific Metals,* L. Friberg, G. F. Nordberg, V. B. Vouk, Eds., Elsevier, Amsterdam, 1986, pp 185-210.

[12]   Hanawa, T., Kaga, M., Itoh, Y., Echizenya, T., Oguchi, H., and Ota, M., Cytotoxicities of Oxides, Phosphates and Sulphides of Metals, *Biomaterials,* Vol. 13, 1992, pp 20-24.

[13]   Urban, R.M., Jacobs, J.J., Tomlinson, M.J., Black, J., Turner, T.M., and Galante, J.O., "Particles of Metal Alloys and Their Corrosion Products in the Liver, Spleen and Para-Aortic Lymph Nodes of Patients with Total Hip Replacement Prostheses," *Transactions of the Orthopaedic Research Society,* Vol. 20, February 1995, p 241.

[14]   Cook, S.D., Barrack, R.L., Clemow, A.J.T., " Corrosion and Wear at the Modular Interface of Uncemented Femoral Stems," *The Journal of Bone and Joint Surgery*, Vol. 76-B, No. 1, January 1994, pp 68-72.

[15]   Collier, J.P., Mayor, M.B., Williams, I.R., Suprenant, V.A., Suprenant, H.P., and Currier, B.H., " The Tradeoffs Associated with Modular Hip Prostheses," *Clinical Orthopaedics and Related Research*, Number 311, February 1995, pp 91-101.

Jeremy L. Gilbert[1] and Joshua J. Jacobs[2]

THE MECHANICAL AND ELECTROCHEMICAL PROCESSES ASSOCIATED WITH TAPER FRETTING CREVICE CORROSION: A REVIEW

REFERENCE: Gilbert, J.L. and Jacobs, J.J., "**The Mechanical and Electrochemical Processes Associated with Taper Fretting Crevice Corrosion: A Review,**" *Modularity of Orthopedic Implants, ASTM STP 1301,* Donald E. Marlowe, Jack E. Parr, and Michael B. Mayor, Eds., American Society for Testing and Materials, 1997.

ABSTRACT: Implant modularity has become a primary implant design concept used in total hip replacement procedures. However, over the last 5 years evidence of corrosion attack in taper crevices formed at the junction of these components has come to light from retrieval analyses. The goals of this paper are to summarize the results of retrieval studies and to discuss the material properties and the mechanical and electrochemical processes which are hypothesized to govern the corrosion attack observed. This paper will review several test methodologies developed by the authors to evaluate aspects of the proposed mechanism of mechanically assisted crevice corrosion. Retrieval studies have shown that both mixed-alloy (Ti-6Al-4V stems and Co-Cr-Mo heads) and similar-alloy (Co-Cr-Mo stems and Co-Cr-Mo heads, and Ti-6Al-4V stems and Ti-6Al-4V heads) couples demonstrate corrosion attack in-vivo. These results indicate that this corrosion process is not due solely to the mixing of dissimilar metals but may occur as a result of mechanical-electrochemical interactions in the taper crevice. Oxide film fracture due to mechanical fretting and the restricted crevice environment of the taper combine to cause changes in the solution chemistry of the fluid inside the taper including pH drops and increases in chloride concentrations. Furthermore, the potential of the implant can become significantly more negative causing the oxide film which reforms to be thinner than the original film and moves the implant's potential toward the active range for corrosion attack. The role of solution chemistry, sample potential and the mechanical tenacity of the oxide films and the test methods used to evaluate these factors will be discussed as they effect the corrosion attack observed.

KEYWORDS: Modularity, corrosion, crevice, fretting, oxide films, Titanium, Cobalt, Chromium

1. Associate Professor, Division of Biological Materials, Northwestern University, Chicago, IL 60611, 2. Associate Professor, Department of Orthopedic Surgery, Rush Presbyterian St. Lukes Medical Center, Chicago, IL 60612.

INTRODUCTION

Implant modularity has become one of the central design features of orthopedic implants. Currently, a majority of total hips and total knee prostheses utilize some aspect of modularity in their design. The main issue of concern (which will be addressed in this paper) is the crevice which is formed at the junction of some modular connections. This paper focuses on femoral total hip replacement components with modular head-neck assemblies. However, the processes to be described may occur at other modular connections where crevices are formed. This modular connection typically consists of a metallic-to-metallic or ceramic-to-metallic tapered conical junction where the head component has a tapered bore and the stem has a tapered cone. These tapers can vary from manufacturer to manufacturer in terms of the cone and bore angles and tolerances, surface roughness, materials used, cone and bore diameter and the presence of skirts. Typically, the materials used in these connections consist of a Co-Cr-Mo head (ASTM F-75 or ASTM F-799) or ceramic head (Al_2O_3, ZrO_2) connected to either a Ti-6Al-4V stem (ASTM F-136) or a Co-Cr-Mo stem (ASTM F-75 or F-799). The taper surfaces which come in contact can be either as-machined, ground or polished.

When these tapered connections are assembled they result in a crevice at the junction. Early corrosion testing of crevice geometries and mixed metal couples did not identify any untoward electrochemical consequences of coupling either Co-Cr-Mo or Ti-6Al-4V to each other or themselves [1-4] . Rostoker[3], however, did present some evidence of tarnishing in a Co-Cr/Titanium couple after 100 days of immersion. Hence, for the most part, a galvanic attack or a crevice corrosion attack was not anticipated to result from these tapered devices.

Retrieval studies starting with Mathiesen and Svennson in the late 1980's [5,6], began to demonstrate corrosion attack in the taper junction. Mathiesen reported on 9 Lord Prostheses (Co-Cr-Mo heads on Co-Cr-Mo stems) and showed that 4 had significant signs of a penetrating, etching type of attack. This group stated that, since there were no signs of fretting evident, this attack was not the result of a fretting corrosion attack. They did, however, report on one case where a fulminant pseudotumor developed in the region of the taper connection which was subsequently shown to contain large amounts of corrosion debris associated with the modular connection [6]. More recently, Collier et al. [7,8], Gilbert et al. [9], Cook et al. [10], and Lieberman et al. [11] reported on the incidence of corrosion attack present in modular femoral hip prostheses retrieved from patients for a wide variety of reasons. Table 1 summarizes these retrieval study results. Typical evidence of corrosion attack included etching, pitting, intergranular attack, selective dissolution of cobalt and fretting corrosion [9]. Collier et al. [7,8] presented results which showed that only mixed taper connections (Co-Cr-Mo heads on Ti-6Al-4V stems, 54%) and not similar alloy connections (Co-Cr-Mo heads on Co-Cr-Mo stems or Ti-6Al-4V heads on Ti-6Al-4V stems) showed any signs of attack within the modular connection. They hypothesized that a combination of crevice, oxide fracture and galvanism resulted in a preferential attack of the Co-Cr-Mo alloy surface within the taper.

Gilbert et al.[9] presented the results of an analysis of 148 retrieved implants and showed that both mixed and similar metal combinations were corroding in upwards of 35% of mixed and 23% of similar metal tapers. In this work, a hypothesis was presented for the mechanism of attack where mechanically assisted crevice corrosion (or fretting crevice corrosion) is taking place.

TABLE 1:   PERCENT OF RETRIEVED IMPLANTS CORRODED

Study	CoCr/CoCr	CoCr/Ti	Ti/Ti
Mathiesen	44	-	-
Collier	0	57	0
Gilbert	23	35	-
Cook	7	35	67

- = did not report

Cook et al. [10] reported on a retrieval pool of 109 implants and also demonstrated that mixed and similar metal connections were subject to the corrosion attack seen. They report that upwards of 35% of mixed and 7% of similar metal (CoCr/CoCr) taper connections in their pool of retrievals show evidence of corrosion and fretting. These authors also speculate as to the mechanism of attack and propose that a combination of galvanism, fretting and crevice corrosion are present.

Lieberman et al. [11] report of the results of a smaller group of modular connections and also speculate that a combination of fretting and crevice corrosion is taking place.

More recently, Urban et al. [12] have shown that fretting crevice corrosion products can be seen egressing from the taper connection in retrieved prostheses, and identified similar particulate debris in the pseudocapsule, the articulating surfaces, and in osteolytic lesions. Jacobs, et al. [13] have also reported increased serum Co and urine Cr ions from patients identified as having moderately or severely corroded prostheses. Gilbert et al. [14] have presented two cases where severely corroded similar metal tapers fractured by a corrosion fatigue process where extensive intergranular corrosion attack in combination with prolonged fatigue loading was identified in Co-Cr-Mo stems. Each of these studies have identified significant clinical ramifications resulting from this fretting crevice corrosion attack in-vivo and point to the overall concern associated with the use of modular taper connections in orthopedic implants.

What has not yet been demonstrated fully are detailed mechanisms which delineate the mechanically assisted corrosion process, what geometric and material parameters are most important in governing its incidence, and ultimately what design, material or surface modifications can be effected to limit or eliminate this process without eliminating the taper connection itself.

The present paper will review in more detail the hypothesis of mechanically assisted crevice corrosion and the testing which we have undertaken to evaluate this process. In our earlier work, we proposed a mechanism of mechanically assisted crevice corrosion (see Fig.

1) which is a modification of the standard theory used to explain crevice corrosion [15]. In the standard mechanism of crevice corrosion, fluid ingress into the taper crevice is followed by corrosion reactions within the crevice which consume the dissolved oxygen in the crevice solution. With continued ionic dissolution, a lack of oxygen then requires that additional chloride ions migrate into the crevice to balance the excess cationic charge and metal chlorides are formed.

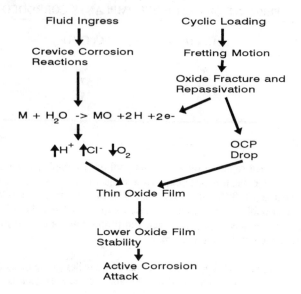

FIGURE 1: Schematic of the Mechanism of Mechanically Assisted Crevice Corrosion

These metal chlorides then have the effect of hydrolyzing water and resulting in a metal oxide (or hydroxide) and hydrochloric acid according to the reaction below

$$M^{n+}Cl_n^- + \frac{n}{2}H_2O \rightarrow MO_{\frac{n}{2}} + nHCl \tag{1}$$

where M^{n+} represents the cationic species involved. The crevice solution then becomes more highly acidic and higher chloride concentration is developed. These combine to accelerate the attack within the crevice and result in an autoaccelerating process.

The rate at which crevice corrosion occurs depends on the rate of several kinetic processes. If O_2 ingress into the crevice is large compared to the rate of ionic dissolution, then crevice corrosion will not occur to any large extent. This is thought to be the case when passivating alloys form crevices, as in orthopedic alloys or when the crevices are large enough to easily exchange fluid with the outside solution. The oxide films which form on the surface inhibit the rate of ionic dissolution thus minimizing the consumption of oxygen and limiting the pH drops and [Cl] rises necessary for accelerated attack.

However, another stimulus which must be considered in the corrosion process of modular taper connections, since these connections are cyclically loaded, is large cyclic stresses and the potential for fretting. Fretting is defined as small scale relative cyclic motion between two objects. Typical fretting distances are between 1 μm and 100 μm. When fretting is present it is possible that the asperity contacts between the two taper surfaces will develop high enough shear and compressive stresses to induce oxide film fracture. That is, the passivating metal oxide film will be abraded by the fretting process. A schematic of how a metal surface repassivates after oxide fracture is shown in Figure 2.

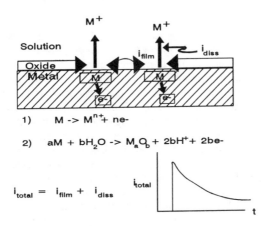

Figure 2: Schematic of oxide repassivation reactions after mechanical disruption. After film disruption, both ionic dissolution and film growth currents are generated.

Oxide fracture will have a significant effect in terms of the corrosion behavior because it exposes underlying unreacted metal which will both increase the rate of ionic dissolution and will also spontaneously reform an oxide film (i.e., repassivate). Because of the high free energies of formation of these oxide films, they will reform utilizing oxygen from just about any source including water itself. That is, repassivation in aqueous solutions will hydrolyze water according to the following reaction.

$$M + H_2O \rightarrow MO + 2H^+ + 2e^- \tag{2}$$

It should be noted that this reaction does not require apriori formation of metal chlorides, but rather forms directly from exposed metal. Chloride ions will migrate into the crevice in this case to balance the H^+ ions generated. This was demonstrated by Ratzer Shiebe [16] in experiments of titanium oxide abrasion and repassivation. In that work, titanium abraded in anhydrous ionic methanol did not exhibit any repassivation currents. However, in the presence of even 1% H_2O, there were significant repassivation currents.

In the presence of fretting, the crevice corrosion mechanism can be significantly altered, dramatically increasing the rates of reaction within the crevice and accelerating the overall attack. Therefore, mechanically assisted crevice corrosion is hypothesized to be the result of the combined attack of mechanical abrasion of the surface oxide films and the chemistry changes which transpire within the crevice solution.

The remainder of this paper will discuss the experiments and test methodologies developed in our laboratory to investigate several aspects of this process. These methods include techniques for monitoring the expected solution chemistry changes in the taper region, monitoring open circuit potential and fretting corrosion currents during cyclic loading, and a scratch test method to evaluate mechanical and electrochemical reactions to controlled high speed disruption of the oxide film.

TEST METHODS

From the above hypothesis, it can be seen that there are several indicators and measures which can be evaluated to assess fretting crevice corrosion. Cyclic loading of tapers in solution, and monitoring the open circuit potential (OCP) and fretting corrosion currents provides a means to determine how cyclic loads affect fretting crevice corrosion. These tests are particularly useful in evaluating the cyclic loads required to initiate fretting crevice corrosion in actual taper connections. With ion specific electrodes for chloride, pH and oxygen, one can monitor solution changes inside the head as a function of time and/or cyclic loading. Long term cyclic loading can be used to generate significant amounts of fretting debris and ionic species both inside the taper crevice and outside which can be measured with a variety of techniques (e.g., atomic absorption spectrometry). Finally, a more basic scratch test of oxide films, immersed in solution and potentiostatically held, can provide highly sensitive and accurate information concerning the effects of fretting contact loads, sample potential and solution conditions on the fretting corrosion reactions associated with oxide fracture and repassivation. The following sections describe these three test methods: 1. the effect of cyclic load on fretting corrosion of tapers, 2. long term testing of tapers and 3. electrochemical scratch testing of oxide films.

Short Term Tests: The effect of cyclic load magnitude on fretting corrosion currents

In the first series of tests, actual femoral tapers are evaluated in-vitro. A taper junction consisting of a stem component and a head component is assembled and immersed in solution (see Fig. 3). Then two electrodes are attached to this sample. The first is a reference electrode which is attached by way of a high impedance voltmeter and the second, a titanium alloy (Ti-6Al-4V) electrode which is connected by way of a zero resistance ammeter. In this way, the (OCP) of the sample and titanium electrode can be monitored (by the voltmeter) while the currents which pass from the sample to the titanium electrode can be measured with the ammeter. Similar approaches have been used by others [17] in the evaluation of modular tapers.

Current will flow between these two electrodes when there is a potential difference between sample and titanium. When fretting occurs at the taper interface, electrons are generated by the hydrolysis reaction of Eq. 2 as repassivation takes place which, in turn, will lower the potential of the sample surface (more negative OCP). The OCP measurement is thus an average OCP for both sample and Ti-electrode, and deviations of OCP from at-rest values will indicate the onset of fretting corrosion. The fretting currents which flow from sample to Ti-electrode are due to this potential difference between sample and Ti-electrode.

The entire assembly is then placed into the load frame of a servohydraulic test machine (Instron model 1350, Canton, MA) in a neutral anatomic orientation and a cyclic

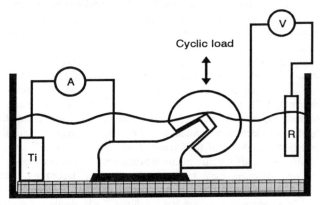

FIGURE 3: Schematic of sample and testing apparatus configuration.

load is applied to the head component of the taper sample. These cyclic loads start at very low values and are periodically incremented to higher and higher values and the OCP and fretting currents are monitored. From this test method, one can obtain several parameters including the load to initiate fretting corrosion and the magnitude of the fretting corrosion at a set load. The load at onset is determined when there is deviation of the OCP, mean fretting current and fretting current amplitude associated with cyclic loading. Figure 4 shows the typical response of a taper during one of these tests. It is interesting to note that the OCP during cyclic loading can drop as much as -500 mV from its rest value. As discussed below, this effect may have ramifications in terms of the oxide film over the entire implant.

This method is able to comparatively evaluate material, design, surface roughness and surface treatment effects on the fretting corrosion performance. It is also able to determine how loading parameters such as magnitude and frequency affect the corrosion process.

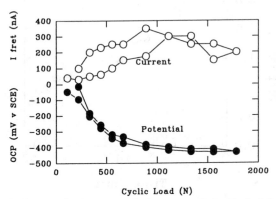

FIGURE 4: OCP and fretting corrosion current magnitude versus applied cyclic load for a mixed couple in phosphate buffered saline.

Long Term Tests

Rest tests--In these series of tests, several parameters can be studied. As outlined above, it is hypothesized that changes will occur in the crevice solution chemistry with crevice corrosion and that the addition of fretting may compound and accelerate these events. Furthermore, analysis of tapers after prolonged cyclic loading under physiological solution conditions can help to elucidate and evaluate specific implant design and material effects.

To evaluate solution chemistry changes, access is gained to the interior of the head by drilling a hole in the head component. A series of ion specific electrodes are sealed in placed to monitor pH, [Cl], and P_{O2} within the crevice solution. To assure that solution contact is maintained, the taper crevice is prefilled with saline prior to assembling the taper. Besides assuring that the electrodes maintain solution contact in the taper, this condition also presents a "worst-case" condition of fluid penetration. To monitor [Cl] and pH, a silver-chlorided silver wire, and a pH specific microelectrode are used, respectively. Both of these electrodes have demonstrated long term stability in our laboratory (several days). Silver/silver chloride electrodes can be made by potentiostatically holding a silver wire at 1.0 to 1.5 V vs SCE in a saturated aqueous NaCl solution. pH electrodes are commercially available (Lazar Inc., Los Angeles, CA). These electrodes measure a potential difference between the ion specific electrode and a reference electrode and, using the Nernst equation, the molar concentration of these ions can be determined. To monitor oxygen, a platinum wire electrode is used with an amperometric technique. In this technique, the Pt electrode is swept through a range of potentials using cyclic voltammetry [18], (CV), then the current at a set negative potential such as -800 mV vs SCE is used as a measure of the oxygen content in the solution. Since oxygen is being reduced by this electrode at these potentials, the magnitude of the current can be directly related to the concentration of O_2 (see Fig. 5). In this figure, the current through the Pt wire is dependent upon the concentration of oxygen in solution. As O_2 is removed by N_2 bubbling, the amperometric current is reduced demonstrating the O_2 dependence on the current.

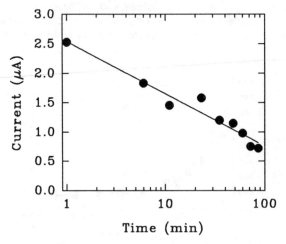

FIGURE 5: Plot of cyclic voltammetry currents in the downward sweep at - 800 mV versus time of bubbling nitrogen gas. As the solution is deaerated, the currents decrease as well.

These methods have been applied to taper geometries, the details of which are reported elsewhere [19-22]. The major findings from this chemistry monitoring is that, even at rest without the application of cyclic load, pH drops, chloride increases and oxygen decreases with time in the solution inside the taper crevice. This result implies that the reactions described above (oxygen consumption, water hydrolysis and chloride ingress) are present and operating in tapers with solution present and no loading. We have shown that, over a time frame of about 48 to 100 hrs, pH drops of two or more units, increases in chloride up to 2 M (from a starting concentration of 0.18 M) and 50% decreases in amperometric measurement of O_2 are found [22]. These results imply that crevices alone provide some driving force for the proposed solution changes even in the absence of mechanical loading. However, little or no corrosion damage is evident optically or microscopically after solution immersion only.

Cyclic Mechanical Loading--In the long term cyclic fretting corrosion tests, a sinusoidal 2000 N load is applied at 5 Hz and a load ratio, R, of 0.1. These tests were performed while the sample is immersed in solution and solution is present in the head. Internal head solution chemistry is periodically monitored and the OCP and fretting currents are monitored as described above. These long term tests required 2.3 days to reach 1 million cycles. After testing, metallic ion levels, particle generation and surface damage can all be assessed to provide measures of the extent of fretting corrosion present. These latter tests have not been performed as yet.

When cyclic loading is applied to these tapers, similar solution changes are observed as compared to the rest tests. At present not enough information has been generated to detect statistical differences between rest and cyclic tests in terms of pH, [Cl] and O_2 changes. However, during cyclic testing out to 1 million cycles of load, it is clear that fretting currents are being generated and OCP is shifting to lower values. During cyclic loading, there is an initial high fretting corrosion current and large OCP shifts to more negative potentials. With time, over about 24 hrs, the OCP slowly recovers to close to the initial potential and the fretting currents diminish. Occasionally, OCP will spontaneously drop and fretting currents will increase. Similarly, if the test is interrupted and then restarted, initially high transients may occur which settle with time. After long term testing we have seen damage to taper surface on Scanning Electron Microscopy [22] which appears to be a combined fretting corrosion attack and crevice corrosion (i.e., mechanically assisted crevice corrosion), similar to but not as extensive as those seen in some retrievals.

Scratch Tests--The last testing methodology the authors have developed to assess the process of oxide fracture and repassivation consists of an electrochemical scratch test [23-25]. In this test, a custom built load cell consisting of a diamond stylus approximately 18 μm in diameter is attached to a calibrated double cantilever system. The load cell consists of two metal strip cantilevers attached to the core of a Linear Variable Differential Transformer (LVDT) which can detect displacements of less than 0.1 μm. The double cantilever allows vertical deflection to deliver controlled loads to the diamond tip, while at the same time providing high rigidity in the lateral directions. This load cell is attached to the high speed piezoelectric actuators of the scanning electrochemical microscope (SECM) [26] which can translate the probe over a surface anywhere from 1 μm to 90 μm in approximately 1 ms [23]. Hence, high speed scratches and controlled loads can be applied through a diamond tip to a surface. Similarly, because the diamond load cell assembly is attached to the movement controls of the SECM, one can use this system to obtain a contact topographic image of the surface after a controlled scratch is applied.

The sample surface can be immersed in a phosphate buffered saline solution and electrochemically controlled using potentiostatic techniques. Then, as the oxide film is disrupted, a current transient associated with the repassivation process is created which can be detected with computer-based data acquisition methods. This technique is described in more detail elsewhere [23-25]. The advantages of this technique are that very controlled loads (to about 0.002 N) and very controlled displacements, and thus scratch areas, can be applied at very high rates. Variations in applied load, solution chemistry, surface preparation or sample potential can be effected and evaluated.

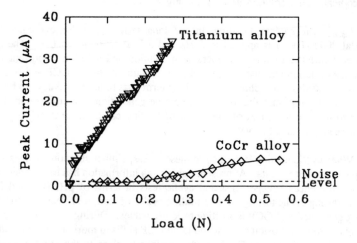

Figure 6: Peak scratch current versus load for both Ti-6Al-4V and Co-Cr-Mo alloy oxides. Note the much larger loads required to induce oxide fracture in Co-Cr-Mo than Ti-6Al-4V.

The results from tests on Ti-6Al-4V and Co-Cr-Mo alloys, reported elsewhere [23-25], have demonstrated several effects. At a set potential of 0 mV SCE, the load-variation tests demonstrated that Ti-6Al-4V can have its oxide film fractured (i.e., current transients are generated) at tip loads as low as 0.002 N, the lower limit of the controlled loading for this system (see Fig. 6). However, for Co-Cr-Mo the load required to initiate oxide film rupture is about 0.25 N. This indicates the relative strength of these oxide films to their substrates. Topographic images of the Ti alloy surface after scratching with different applied loads showed that the lowest applied load to induce detectable permanent surface deformation was about 0.05 N. This implies that titanium oxide film fracture can occur even in the absence of permanent substrate deformation. For Co-Cr-Mo, however, the same experiment showed that permanent surface deformation occurs at 0.25 N, roughly the same load where current transients were detected. Thus, Co-Cr alloy oxide films will not fracture or abrade until the local alloy substrate is deformed permanently.

Sample potential has a systematic effect on the peak currents and time constants for repassivation during these scratch tests when the scratch length and applied load are constant (see Fig. 7). For pH 7 saline, at negative potentials (between -900 and -500 mV SCE) for both titanium and Co-Cr alloys, there are little or no current transients detected. As the potential is increased, current transients begin to appear at about -800 mV for Ti-6Al-4V and -450 mV for Co-Cr-Mo (see Fig. 7). Peak currents increase approximately linearly with applied potential in both alloy systems. For Co-Cr alloys, these peak currents increase, reaching a maximum at about +300 mV and then decrease as the alloy begins to enter the transpassive region for this material. For Ti-6Al-4V the peak currents continue to increase up through 1000 mV. There are small but statistically significant effects of solution aeration, and pH on the slope of the peak current versus potential curves for Ti-6Al-4V while the results from Co-Cr-Mo tests did not show significant differences. Even, with these differences, the actual peak current magnitudes at a set potential for the different solution conditions show only small differences. There is an effect of pH on the potential at onset and the time constants for repassivation. Solutions with a pH of 2 appear to have slower repassivation time constants in the potential region of 0 to -500 mV compared to pH 7 solutions. Time constants ranged from 0.5 ms to 2.5 ms depending on potential, solution pH and material. The potential for onset of current transients increased for Ti-6Al-4V from about -800 to -500 as pH went from 7 to 2.

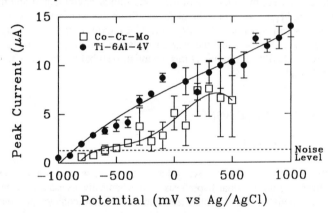

Figure 7: Peak current versus potential for Ti-6Al-4V and Co-Cr-Mo in physiological saline. Note the higher potentials required to initiate a current transient for Co-Cr-Mo. 30 μm scratch, Loads = 0.1 N for Ti and 0.35 N for Co-Cr-Mo.

In a previous publication [23], we have proposed a model to describe the repassivation behavior in terms of the kinetics of oxide film regrowth and the ionic dissolution process which occurs through the exposed metal surface. Adapting the model proposed by Ambrose [27], in which a first order differential equation governing the surface area fraction covered by oxide film at any time after removal of the oxide is developed, and solving the resultant differential equation using an exponential forcing function for the current transient (as is observed experimentally), we found that the peak current, I_p, is given by

$$I_p - \frac{\delta \rho n F A_o}{MW\tau} + j_o A_o \exp[\frac{\eta}{b_a}]$$

where δ = oxide film thickness, n is the valence of the cation, F is the Faraday constant, ρ is the density, MW is the molecular weight, τ is the time constant for repassivation, j_o is the exchange current density, η is the over potential, A_o is the exposed area, and b_a is the Tafel constant for ionic dissolution. The second term is related to ionic dissolution from the exposed metal surface and may or may not be significant depending on the ionic reactions possible and their overpotential. In this equation, the oxide film thickness, δ, is assumed to be constant during repassivation (for a constant potential) and that the oxide film grows over the entire exposed surface. It has been shown that the oxide film thickening rate is potential dependent and that for titanium an oxide film thickening rate of 2 nm/V has been reported [28,29]. This implies that the oxide film which reforms after abrasion will depend on the potential of the surface. The more negative the potential (i.e., closer to the equilibrium potential), the thinner will be the oxide film. Hence, this analysis can result in a measure of the film thickening rate, the thickness of the oxide film at any potential and the potential where the oxide film begins to form or breakdown. From these observations, it can be seen that titanium oxides can form at -800 mV while CoCr oxides start at -450 to -500 mV. Another observation of interest is that the peak currents begin to drop at +300 for Co-Cr-Mo indicating that the oxide film is thinning at this potential, well before the breakdown potential of 550 mV for this alloy.

DISCUSSION AND CONCLUSIONS

<u>Modifications to the Hypothesis</u>

From the results of the above described tests, there are several comments which need to be made concerning the original hypothesis of mechanically assisted crevice corrosion. First, in the initial model, it was hypothesized that the solution changes proposed to occur during crevice corrosion, would not develop without the presence of mechanical fretting. However, the rest tests monitoring solution chemistry found that, if solution is present inside the crevice, it experiences decreases in pH and increases in [Cl] with time. These observations imply that mechanical loading is not a prerequisite for some level of crevice corrosion to occur in these tapers. The extent of change in solution chemistry may not, however, be sufficient to cause the autocatalytic changes seen in the classic model of crevice corrosion.

Second, the short term tests of taper samples have shown that the loads to initiate fretting are low compared to the physiological loads to be expected in these devices. Thus, the tapers will most likely experience fretting corrosion when the patient loads his/her prosthesis. These fretting reactions act to decrease the potential of the entire implant (i.e., make more negative). This may well have the effect of thinning the oxide film which reforms in the crevice after abrasion, and may also thin the oxide film elsewhere on the implant surface. The in-vitro tests of tapers showed that at 2000 N, the potential of the implant can reach -500 mV which is approximately where no oxide fracture and repassivation current transients are detected for Co-Cr-Mo scratch tests and only small transients are seen for titanium. Hence, the oxide films in these taper regions are most likely thinner than would be expected with no load and thus provide less of a barrier to ion release. These potentials are high enough, however, to be well above the equilibrium potential for anodic reactions of the underlying metal ion and hence it is to be expected that some accelerated corrosion will occur. With cycling during long term testing, the potentials tend to recover over time. This implies a decrease in fretting corrosion reactions. As pointed out by Smith and Ducheyne [30], this may be due to the accumulation of fretting corrosion debris in the taper which may act like a boundary lubricant between surfaces.

Third, the loads (or stresses) required to cause oxide fracture as determined from the scratch tests are significantly greater for Co-Cr-Mo surfaces, than for Ti-6Al-4V. These scratch loads for titanium most likely facilitate the fretting crevice corrosion process for mixed tapers compared to similar taper couples because of the ease of titanium oxide fracture during the fretting process and the magnitude of the repassivation currents generated. Hence one might speculate that the apparent increase in rates of corrosion in the taper might be attributed to the relative ease of oxide fracture of titanium oxide compared to Co-Cr-Mo oxide. However, titanium typically does not show the extensive corrosion attack seen in Co-Cr-Mo because of the greater range of potential and pH where its oxide is stable, whereas, Co-Cr-Mo oxides have a smaller range of pH and potential for stability. Lowering pH and potential (as seen in these experiments) can put the Co-Cr-Mo into an active state (i.e., where anodic dissolution can occur without oxide film formation) which can lead to the etching and other forms of corrosion attack observed.

From these observations, the mechanisms of mechanically assisted crevice corrosion may have to be modified as follows. Fluid ingress into the taper crevice and the presence of the crevice alone appears to significantly alter the crevice solution chemistry in much the same way as the standard crevice corrosion model proposes. However, these changes are inadequate by themselves to autocatalyze the crevice corrosion process. Taper fretting crevice corrosion is induced in modular tapers when they are loaded at physiological levels. All tapers tested to date in our laboratory consisting of native metal-oxide surfaces exhibit fretting corrosion currents and changes in OCP with cyclic loading at loads well below those expected physiologically. Thus, fretting corrosion is most likely present in these tapers. Fretting results in oxide fracture and repassivation processes which hydrolyze water to form metal oxide and hydrogen ions. Chloride ions can then migrate into the crevice to balance the hydrogen ions. With lower pH and increased [Cl] repassivation time constants increase slowing the oxide reformation rate, and lower potentials thin the oxide that reforms making it less capable of resisting corrosion attack.

It is hypothesized that all of these changes ultimately promote a crevice environment which is acidic, high [Cl], and deaerated. Furthermore, the metal-oxide on the surface is thinner and less able to resist attack ultimately resulting in the large scale etching and other localized corrosion features seen in the retrieved implants

ACKNOWLEDGEMENTS: Aspects of these studies have been supported by Osteonics, Inc., Zimmer, Inc.

REFERENCES
1.   Griffin, CD, Buchanan, RA, Lemmons, JE, "*In-vitro* Electrochemical Corrosion Study of Coupled Surgical Implant Materials", J. Biomed. Mater. Res., Vol. 17, 1983, pp 489-500.
2.   Lucas, LC, Buchanan, RA, Lemons, JE, "Investigations on the Galvanic Corrosion of Multialloy Total Hip Prostheses", J. Biomed. Mater. Res., Vol. 15, 1981, pp 731-747.
3.   Rostoker, W, Pretzel, CW, Galante, JO, "Couple Corrosion Among Alloys for Skeletal Prostheses", J. Biomed. Mater. Res., Vol. 8, 1974, pp 407-419.
4.   Jacobs, JJ, Latanision, RM Rose, RM, Veeck, SJ, "The Effect of Porous Coatings Processing on the Corrosion Behavior of Cast Co-Cr-Mo Surgical Implant Alloy", J. Orthop. Res., Vol. 8, No. 6, 1990, pp 874-882.
5.   Mathiesen, EB, Lindgren, JU, Blomgren, GGA, Reinholt, FP, "Corrosion of Modular Hip Prostheses", J. Bone and Joint Surgery, Vol. 73-B, 1991, pp 569-575.
6.   Svennson, O, Mathiesen, EB, Reinholt, FP, Blomgren, GA, "Formation of a Fulminant Soft Tissue Pseudotumor after Uncemented Hip Arthroplasty", J. Bone and Joint Surgery, 70A, 1238-1242, 1988.
7.   Collier, JP, Surprenant, VA, Jensen, RE, Mayor, MB, "Corrosion at the Interface of Cobalt-Alloy Heads On Titanium-Alloy Stems", Clin. Orthop. and Rel. Res., No 271, 1991, pp 305-312.
8.   Collier, JP, Surprenant, VA, Jensen, RE, Mayor, MB, Surprenant, HE, "Corrosion Between The Components of Modular Femoral Hip Prostheses", J. Bone and Joint Surgery, Vol. 74-B, 1992, pp 511-517.
9.   J.L. Gilbert, C.A. Buckley, J.J. Jacobs, "In-Vivo Corrosion of Modular Hip Prosthesis Components in Mixed and Similar Metal Combinations: The Effect of Crevice, Stress, Motion and Alloy Coupling", J. Biomed. Mater. Res., Vol. 27, No. 12, pp 1533-1544, (1993).
10.   Cook, SD, Barrack, RL, Clemow, AJT, "Corrosion and Wear at the Modular Interface of Uncemented Femoral Stems", J Bone and Joint Surgery, Vol. 76-B, No. 1, 1994, pp 68-72.
11.   Lieberman, J.R., Rimnac, C.M., Garvin, K.L. Klein, R.W., and Salvati, E.A., "An Analysis of the Head-Neck Taper Interface in Retrieved Hip Prostheses", Clin. Ortho. and Rel. Res., Vol. 300, March 1994, pp 162-167.
12.   R. Urban, J.J. Jacobs, J.L. Gilbert, J.O. Galante, "Migration of Corrosion Products from Modular Hip Prostheses. Particle Microanalysis and Histopathological Findings", J. Bone and Joint Surgery, Vol. 76-A, No. 9, September 1994, pp 1345-1359.
13.   J.J. Jacobs, R.M. Urban, J.L. Gilbert, A.K. Skipor, J. Black, M. Jasty, J.O. Galante, "Local and Distant Products From Modularity", Hip Society Meeting, Clin. Orthopedics and Rel. Res., Vol. 319, 1995, pp 94-105.
14.   J.L. Gilbert, J.J. Jacobs, C.A. Buckley, K.C. Bertin, M. Zernich, "Intergranular Corrosion Fatigue Failure of Co-Cr Femoral Stems: A Failure Analysis of Two Implants", J. Bone and Joint Surgery, Vol. 76-A, No. 1, January, 1994, pp 110-115.
15.   Fontana, M.G., Greene, D.N., Corrosion Engineering, McGraw-Hill Book Co., NY, 1978.
16.   Ratzer-Schiebe, HJ, "Repassivation of Titanium and Titanium Alloys Dependent on Potential and pH", Passivity of Metals and Semiconductors, Ed. M. Froment,

Elsevier Science, Amsterdam, 1981, pp. 731-739.

17.   Brown, S.A., Flemming, C.A.C., Kawalec, J.S., Placko, H.E., Vassaux, C., Merritt, K, Payer, J.H., Kraay, M.J., "Fretting Corrosion Accelerates Crevice Corrosion of Modular Hip Tapers", J. Applied Biomaterials, Vol. 6, 1995, pp 19-26.

18.   Bard, A.J., Faulkner, L.R., Electrochemical Methods: Fundamentals and Applications, J. Wiley and Sons, New York, 1980.

19.   C.A. Buckley, J.L. Gilbert, "Mechancially Induced Electrochemical Events in Cyclically Loaded Modular Hp Protheses", Trans. of Soc. for Biomaterials, Vol. 17, Boston, 1994, pp 57.

20.   J.L. Gilbert, C.A. Buckley, "Mechanical-Electrochemical Interactions During In-Vitro Fretting Corrosion Tests of Modular Taper Connections", Total Hip Revision Surgery, J.O. Galante A.G. Rosenberg, J.J. Callaghan, ed., Raven Press, New York, 1994, pp 41-50.

21.   JL Gilbert, CA Buckley, JJ Jacobs, EP Lautenschalger, "In-Vitro Mechanical-Electrochemical Testing of the Fretting Corrosion Process in Modular Femoral Tapers", Transaction of Orthopedic Research Society, Vol. 20, 1995 pp 240.

22.   J.R. Goldberg, C.A. Buckley, J.J. Jacobs, J.L. Gilbert, "Corrosion Testing of Modular Implants", Modularity of Orthopedic Implants, ASTM STP 1301, J.E. Parr, M.B. Mayor, D.E. Marlow, Eds., American Socienty for Testing and Materials, Philadelphia, PA, 1996.

23.   JL Gilbert, CA Buckley, EP Lautenschlager, "Titanium Oxide Fracture and Repassivation: The Effect of Potential, pH and Aeration", Medical Applications of Titanium and Its Alloys: The Materials and Biological Issues, ASTM Special Technical Publication 1272, Ed. S.A. Brown, J.E. Lemons, in press 1996.

24.   CA Buckley, JL Gilbert "The Mechanical-Electrochemical Interactions of Passivating Alloys Used in Medicine", Compatibility of Biomedical Implants, Ed. P Kovacs, N Istephanous, Proceedings of the Electrochemical Society, Vol. 94-15, 1994, pp 319-330.

25.   J Goldberg, JL Gilbert, EP Lautenschlager, "Electrochemical Response of Co-Cr-Mo Alloy to Mechanical Disruption of its Passive Oxide Film", Trans. of Soc. for Biomat., Vol. 18, 1995 pp 206.

26.   J.L. Gilbert, S.M. Smith, E.P. Lautenschlager, "Scanning Electrochemical Microscopy of Metallic Biomaterials: Reaction Rate and Ion Release Imaging Modes", J. Biomed. Mat. Res., Vol. 27, No. 11, 1993, pp 1357-1366.

27.   Ambrose, J. R., "Repassivation Kinetics", in Treatise on Materials Science and Technology, Corrosion: Aqueous Processes and Passive Films Ed. JC Scully, Academic Press, NY, 1983, pp 175-204.

28.   Shams, El Din, AM, Hammond, AA, "Oxide Film Formation and Thickness on Titanium in Water", Thin Solid Films, 167, 1988, pp 269-280.

29.   Aladjem, A., "Review: Anodic Oxidation of Titanium and its Alloys", J. Mater. Sci., Vol. 8, 1973, pp 688-704.

30.   Smith, B.J., Ducheyne, P., "Fretting Corrosion of Ti-6Al-4V Reveals Two Fretting Regimes", Trans. Soc. for Biomat., 1994, pp 265.

Jeffrey J. Shea[1], Richard D. Lambert[2], Terry W. McLean[3]

WEAR OF NON-ARTICULATING SURFACES IN MODULAR ACETABULAR CUPS

REFERENCE: Shea, J. J., Lambert, R. D., and McLean, T. W., "Wear of Non-Articulating Surfaces in Modular Acetabular Cups," *Modularity of Orthopedic Implants, ASTM STP 1301,* Donald E. Marlowe, Jack E. Parr, and Michael B. Mayor, Eds., American Society for Testing and Materials, 1997.

ABSTRACT: As a result of histological studies, there have been new developments in the field of modular acetabular cup design. Osteolysis has been isolated as one of the major causes of aseptic loosening of the femoral component in total hip arthroplasty (THA). Histological studies of retrieved tissue during revision THA have revealed a high content of polyethylene (PE) particles which are submicron in size in the surrounding tissue of the loose femoral component. The source of the polyethylene can be easily traced to the liner in the acetabular component. Great efforts have been made in reducing PE wear at the femoral head/liner interface through the use of ceramics, better CoCr polishing techniques, and improved processing of polyethylene. Until recently, however, not much attention has been given to the liner outside diameter/shell inside diameter interface, sometimes known as the "second articulating surface". The first aspect of this paper provides background on various studies which examined metal shell/polyethylene liner interfaces of several commercially available acetabular components. Movement of the liner was confirmed and measured. Various types of surface abrasion were noted on the liners. The second aspect of this paper examines two modular adjunctive fixation methods for debris generation potential. Recommendations for design improvements are included.

KEY WORDS: total hip arthroplasty, osteolysis, PE wear debris, liner lock mechanism, micromotion, interface, adjunctive fixation, metal ion release

Modularity in acetabular cup design was first introduced by Harris in 1971 [1]. The introduction of this device appeared to be a temporary solution to the increasing problem of excessive High Density Polyethylene (HDP) wear rates. Although the use of HDP as a bearing surface was a great improvement over polytetrafluorethylene (PTFE), its performance was still far from ideal. Charnley reported in-vivo wear rates to be 0-1mm in 5 years.[2] Harris hypothesized that modularity would increase the overall longevity of the implant by allowing replacement of the HDP component which was affected by wear the most. The outer metal shell could remain permanently fixed in bone cement without the surgeon performing the typical intrusive removal process associated with revision surgery.

---

[1]Senior Product Development Engineer, Smith & Nephew Richards, Memphis, TN 38116
[2]Senior Research Engineer, Smith & Nephew Richards, Memphis, TN 38116
[3]Senior Research Technician, Smith & Nephew Richards, Memphis, TN 38116

Modularity offered an entire new array of options. Advantages included customization of the patient's implant such as the variability of femoral head size to maximize polyethylene thickness and range of motion, availability of lipped vs. standard liners to help reduce the incidence of dislocation, and the reduction of inventory which otherwise had to be maintained in order to accommodate these options. The main disadvantage recognized with this design was decreased polyethylene thickness which in most cases, was not perceived as a concern. Modularity between the liner and shell also lead to the introduction of threaded acetabular components as well as po⁻ᵘs ingrowth cups which utilized various adjunctive fixation methods - namely cancellous and cortical screws, modular spikes and screws.

Several years after the introduction of modular polyethylene inserts, higher wear rates at the femoral head/liner interface were observed with the two piece devices than the previously used all-polyethylene cups [3]. The reduction in range of motion as the femoral head wore medially in the polyethylene and the eventual "wear through" of the head to the metal backing of the shell were considered to be the pitfalls of the design [1]. Significant advancements have been made in an effort to reduce the wear of modern prosthetic designs through the use of ceramic heads, improved polishing techniques for CoCr heads, and stronger and thicker polyethylene.

Until recently, the effects of wear were considered to be only mechanical and not histological. Polyethylene debris among other things has been identified as one of the primary contributors to osteolysis (formally thought to be "cement disease") [4]. Progressive osteolysis has been well documented clinically by Harris and others [5][6]. P. Campbell's histological studies, among others, have identified submicron sized PE particles in retrieved tissue surrounding loose femoral components during revision THA [7][8].

The additional attention which has been given to the femoral head/liner wear issue has also lead to increased awareness of debris generation in other areas such as the interface between the polyethylene liner and the metal shell. Several studies have been published recently which examined the motion that occurred at the interface and the potential for debris generation. Lieberman et al. examined deformation patterns and frictional torque in modular acetabular liners [9]. Surface abrasion of the liners was measured on five commercially available acetabular components after the cups were mounted at 23° from the horizontal and axially loaded from 222.5N to 2225N for 10 million cycles. Liners were gold coated to enhance the visualization of wear and deformation patterns. Frictional force measurements were also obtained prior to the start of the test and at 2 million cycle increments thereafter. At 890N of joint load and after 10 million cycles, frictional torque values ranged from 6.4N·m to 12.5N·m. All liners showed evidence of abrasion ranging from 1-30% of the convex surface of the liner. Three modes of damage were identified. Those included burnishing, punch out, and gouging. Lieberman's design recommendations were to have a smooth shell ID, a stable liner locking mechanism, smooth edges around screw holes, and no sharp edges at the liner lock mechanism.

Chen et al. directed a study regarding Ultra High Molecular Weight Polyethylene (UHMWPE) wear debris in modular acetabular prostheses [10]. Relative motion of the liner was measured in a effort to assess UHMWPE wear debris production at the interface between the metal shell and liner of 5 commercially available acetabular components. Liners were subjected to long term simultaneous sinusoidal and static loading (10^7 cycles at 3Hz with ±2.5N·m and 220N static load). Wide variations of the liner lock security, wear patterns of the liners, damage sites, and the amount of UHMWPE debris on the shell and liner surfaces were noted. Measured rotational micromotion ranged from 0.96° to undetectable. Average liner surface area wear range was 0.26cm^2-4.61cm^2. Chen's design recommendations, like Lieberman's, included a stable locking mechanism and a smooth shell inside diameter finish to minimize polyethylene liner wear and debris production.

Williams et al. studied the fixation of UHMWPE liners to metal-backed acetabular shells [11]. Seven commercially available acetabular cups were evaluated. The cups were mounted with a 25° inferior-superior tilt. Compressive axial loads from 272-2720N and internal-external torsional loads from ±7.5N·m were applied at a frequency of 10Hz for 10 million cycles. Three linear variable displacement transducers (LVDTs) were mounted in strategic locations to measure rim micromotion, rim subsidence, rotational micromotion, interface slippage, dome micromotion, and dome subsidence. A mean wear score was assigned to each of the components for comparison. Williams concluded that the liner locking mechanisms can break down under physiological and extreme loading conditions, causing motion of the UHMWPE that results in outer surface wear. Williams also emphasized the importance of a tight, durable peripheral lock mechanism.

Modularity between the liner and shell also offered surgeons the option of using cancellous or cortical screws to more rigidly affix porous coated or hydroxylapatite coated shells to the acetabulum in the 1980's. The most popular surgical technique during that time period was a line-to-line fit between the acetabulum and the prosthesis which required the use of screws to stabilize the cup. Some potential problems identified with screws used in this manner were the loosening of the cup during tightening of screws, possible stress shielding, and resulting motion between the metal shell and screws due to cup migration [12]. Modern techniques include press fitting the prosthesis into the acetabulum so that initial stability can be assessed interoperatively [13]. In this case, the surgeon may elect to use only one screw or none at all.

Evidence of screw head abrasion on convex liner surfaces and the shell has been well documented by Bobyn and Collier [12][14]. Alternatives to acetabular screw fixation include fixed spikes, modular spikes, and modular pegs. The advantages of these options are they virtually eliminate the possibility of interface contact with the UHMWPE liner, and metal debris generation and fretting are drastically reduced. The purpose of this study was to provide a comparative analysis of metal debris generation associated with acetabular screws vs. modular pegs. The acetabular screws were tested in the traditional manner (inserted through the cup ID and threaded into host bone). Modular pegs were also inserted through the cup ID but were fixed to the shell by means of a taper or interference fit.

EXPERIMENTAL METHODS:

A 56mm diameter shell (Reflection V, Smith & Nephew Richards, Memphis, TN) and 25mm cancellous screw were removed from sterile packaging. A 4mm diameter hole was drilled in a 2.54cm x 2.54cm x 1.27cm foam simulated bone (Last-A-Foam®, General Plastics Manufacturing Co.,

Tacoma, WA) per normal surgical technique and the screw was assembled
through the shell inside diameter (ID) and screwed into the foam in the
traditional manner per the recommended surgical technique [15]. A
UHMWPE liner was then removed from sterile packaging and assembled in
the shell. The entire shell/screw/liner assembly was placed in an
acetel resin fixture/environmental chamber which positioned the screw at
10° from the vertical. The environmental chamber was then filled with
650ml of Ringer's solution. The chamber was fixed to a servohydraulic
test frame and covered with a polymer shrink wrap for contamination
prevention. The load was applied to the tip of the screw via. an acetel
resin rod (Fig. 1). A sinusoidal compressive load of 44.5-445N was
applied at a rate of 10Hz for 10 million cycles. Upon completion of the
10 million cycles, 25ml of the solution from the chamber was removed and
analyzed by Teledyne Wah Chang (TWC) (Albany, OR) to determine the metal
ion concentration using the Direct Current Plasma/Optical Emission
Spectroscopy method. Precautions were taken to minimize air
contamination. After an initial post test visual inspection, the liners
were gold sputter coated for scanning electron micrograph (SEM)
analysis. This method highlighted details of screw head indentions in
the liner. This experiment was performed 3 times.

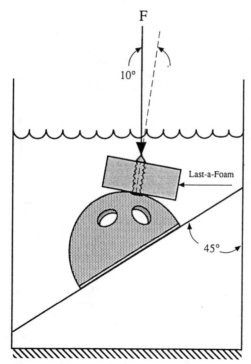

FIG. 1--Schematic of screw fatigue set up.

Next, a 56mm diameter shell (Reflection V) and 15mm modular peg were removed from sterile packaging, foam block prepared, and the peg was impacted in the shell per the recommended surgical technique [15]. The entire fixture/environmental chamber was assembled in the same manner as the screw test set up (Fig. 2). Upon completion of 10 million cycles, 25ml of the solution was again sent to TWC for measurement of metal ion concentration. UHMWPE liners were gold sputter coated for SEM analysis. This experiment was performed 3 times.

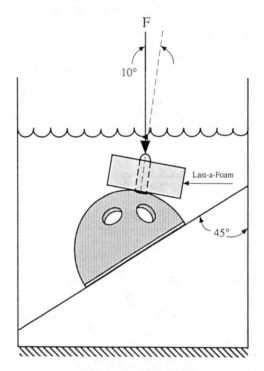

FIG. 2--Schematic of peg fatigue set up.

RESULTS:

Three screws and three pegs were tested. All six of the specimens survived 10 million cycles of fatigue loading. Fig. 3 shows a comparison of the average release of titanium and vanadium ions for screws versus pegs after 10 million cycles. After fatigue testing, all convex surfaces of liners were examined for signs of screw head or peg imprints. Black debris was observed on liners from cups in which screws had been tested (Fig. 4). A black debris "dusting" was also visible on most of the internal surfaces of the environmental chamber once the fluid was removed. Scanning electron micrograph analysis highlighted "half moon" indentions from head contact in all liners where screws were tested (Fig. 5). No debris or indentions were visible on liners from cups in which pegs were evaluated.

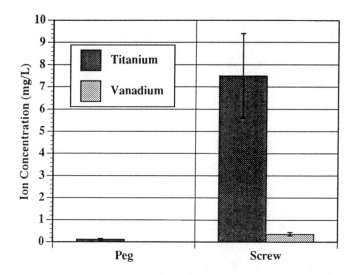

FIG. 3--Average metal ion release of modular pegs vs. screws after 10
million cycles of fatigue loading.

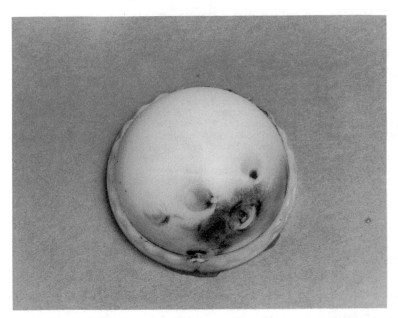

FIG. 4--Metal particulate debris on convex surface of polyethylene
liner.

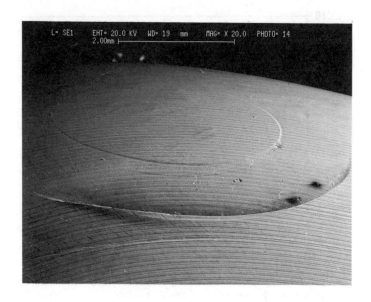

FIG. 5--"Half moon" indention on convex surface of polyethylene
liner from screw head contact.

CONCLUSIONS:

Modularity in porous acetabular components offers many benefits and
options for the surgeon and patient. Modular PE liners are beneficial
in that the surgeon can customize the patient's prosthesis in areas of
femoral head size, PE thickness, and adjunctive fixation for the metal
shell. As more information becomes available regarding the histological
effects of particulate debris, an increased effort should also be made
to minimize debris generation at modular component interfaces.
Lieberman, Chen, and Williams all identified localized areas of back
side wear in their studies by gold sputter coating the convex surfaces
of the liners before testing and macroscopically examining them after
testing. All three authors emphasized the importance of having a stable
liner locking mechanism. Additionally, Lieberman recommended smooth
surfaces on all metal contact areas including the shell inside diameter,
edges around screw holes, and the liner locking mechanism. Chen also
recommended a smooth inside diameter of the shell to minimize
polyethylene debris production.

Methods of adjunctive fixation such as screws, spikes, and pegs need to
be evaluated for potential debris generation. In this study, the
average titanium ion and vanadium ion release for off-axis loading of
screws was 7.5mg/l and 0.36mg/l respectively. The average titanium ion
and vanadium ion release for off-axis loading of modular pegs was

0.12mg/l and <0.05mg/l respectively. Based on the test results from this experiment, one postulation could be that the use of acetabular screws for adjunctive fixation during THA drastically increases the probability of metal ion release and potential for UHMWPE debris generation from screw head abrasion of the liner as the acetabular component moves through its normal subsidence during bone remodeling. The use of modular pegs reduces metal ion release associated with screw usage and decreases the chances for UHMWPE debris generation from head abrasion against the liner.

REFERENCES:

[1]   Harris, W. H., "A New Total Hip Implant," Clinical Orthopedics and Related Research, 1971:81:105-113.

[2]   Charnley, J., "Total Hip Replacement by Low Friction Arthroplasty," Clinical Orthopaedics and Related Research, 1970:72:7-21.

[3]   Cates, H. E., Faris, P. M., Keating, E. M., and Ritter, M. A., "Polyethylene Wear in Cemented Metal-Backed Acetabular Cups," The Journal of Bone and Joint Surgery, Vol. 75-B, No. 2, March 1993, pp 249-253.

[4]   Amstutz, H. C., Campbell, P., Kossovsky, N., and Clarke, I. C., "Mechanism and Clinical Significance of Wear Debris-Induced Osteolysis," Clinical Orthopaedics and Related Research, 1992:276:7-18.

[5]   Harris, W. H. and Schiller, A. C., "Extensive Localized Bone Resorption in the Femur Following Total Hip Replacement," Journal of Bone and Joint Surgery, 58A:612, 1976.

[6]   Schmalzried, T. P., "The Role of High Density Polyethylene in Acetabular Component Loosening," Orthopaedic Research Society, Washington, D.C., 1992.

[7]   Campbell, P. A., Chun, G., Kossovsky, N., and Amstutz, H. C., "Histological Analysis of Tissues Suggests That Metallosis May Really be Plasticosis," 38th Annual Meeting, Orthopaedic Research Society, Washington, D.C., 1992.

[8]   Schmalzried, T. P., Jasty, M., Rosenberg, A., and Harris, W. H., "Histologic Identification of Polyethylene Wear Debris Using Oil Red O Stain," Journal of Applied Biomaterials, 1993, 4: 119-125.

[9]   Lieberman, J. R., Kay, R. M., Hamlet, W., and Kabo, J. M., "Deformation Patterns and Frictional Torque in Modular Acetabular Liners," American Academy of Orthopedic Surgeons, New Orleans, LA, 1994.

[10] Chen, P. C., Mead, E. H., Pinto, J. G., and Colwell, C. W., "Polyethylene Wear Debris in Modular Acetabular Prosthesis," Clinical Orthopedics and Related Research, 1995,:317:44-56.

[11] Williams, V. G., White, S. E., and Whiteside, L. A., "Fixation of Ultra High Molecular Weight Polyethylene Liners to Metal-Backed Acetabular Shells," American Academy of Orthopedic Surgeons, Orlando, FL, 1995.

[12] Bobyn, J. D., Collier, J. P., Mayor, M. B., McTighe, T., Tanzer, M., and Vaughn, B. K., "Particulate Debris in Total Hip Arthroplasty: Problems and Solutions," American Academy of Orthopedic Surgeons, San Francisco, CA, 1993.

[13] Adler, E., Stuchin, S. A., and Kummer, F. J., "Stability of Press-Fit Acetabular Cups," The Journal of Arthroplasty, Vol. 7, No. 3., September 1992, pp 295-301.

[14] Collier, J. P., Mayor, M.B., Jensen, R. E., Suprenant, V. A.,
      Surprenant, H. P., McNamara, J. L., and Belec, L., "Mechanisms of
      Failure of Modular Prostheses," Clinical Orthopaedics and Related
      Research, 1992:285:129-139.
[15] Smith & Nephew Richards Surgical Technique - Reflection I & V
      Porous Coated Acetabular Component, Catalog No. 7138-0127, 1995.

Bernard J. Calès [1]

MARKING OF CERAMIC FEMORAL HEADS

REFERENCE: Calès, B. J., "**Marking of Ceramic Femoral Heads,**" *Modularity of Orthopedic Implants, ASTM STP 1301,* Donald E. Marlowe, Jack E. Parr, and Michael B. Mayor, Eds., American Society for Testing and Materials, 1997.

ABSTRACT: In order to guarantee long term traceability for hip joint heads, permanent marking must be used. Two marking techniques are currently used today for ceramic femoral heads: mechanical machining and laser beam engraving. The objective of this paper was to analyze the risks and advantages of each technique and to evaluate the influence of marking on the mechanical performance of ceramic heads. It has been noted that: -i) the flaws due to mechanical marking are two orders of magnitude larger than for laser engraving, -ii) the stress concentration at the bottom of the head, where machined marking is preferably made, could be significantly higher than at the top of the bore, where laser engraving is currently performed. It is therefore argued that laser engraving is a more suitable marking procedure to guarantee long term reliability.

KEYWORDS: femoral heads, ceramic materials, marking, mechanical properties, stress concentrations.

Ceramic material has been successfully introduced for hip joint head manufacturing for about 20 years [1,2], first Alumina then Zirconia ceramics. These materials are very well accepted as about 175,000 to 200,000 ceramic femoral heads are implanted each year throughout the world. This represents 20% of the total femoral heads produced worldwide.

The reason for the large acceptance of ceramic hip joint heads lies in the reduced UHMWPE wear rate when compared to hip prostheses with metallic heads [3]. Such a polythylene wear rate reduction has been observed in tests on joint simulators and in clinical results [4-6].

Compared to metals, ceramic materials are also characterized by a brittle type fracture. Indeed, the absence of any plasticity for ceramics makes these materials more sensitive to structural flaws or to stress concentrations. For these reasons, control of flaws during ceramic head manufacturing is a key issue for long term reliability and has been extensively investigated by manufacturers.

---

[1]Doctor, Head of R & D, Céramiques Techniques Desmarquest, Z.I. n°1, 27025 Evreux Cedex, France.

In order to guarantee long term traceability for these components permanent marking must be used, as required in appropriate standards, such as ISO 6018 (*Surgical Implants-General Requirements for Marking, Packaging and labelling*) or ASTM F 983-86 (*Standard Practice for Permanent Marking of Orthopaedic Components*). Marking should not compromise the performance of the ceramic head and must be legible over the anticipated service life. Marking is made directly on the heads and must be considered as a potential source of structural flaws. Marking can have direct consequences on ceramic head reliability, if not performed in optimized conditions. Therefore, the marking operation and location must be carefully defined.

Two marking techniques are currently used today for ceramic heads traceability: mechanical machining and laser beam engraving. Two different locations are usually chosen to engrave the required information on the product. The objective of this paper is to analyze the risks and advantages of each technique and to evaluate the influence of marking on the mechanical performance of ceramic heads.

MICROSTRUCTURAL CONSEQUENCE OF MARKING

Mechanical Marking

Marking of ceramic femoral heads using mechanical machining is usually performed when the parts are in the green (pre-sintered) stage. This is done with the help of very fine tools (drills or needle-punches). Marking consists of small grooves making number or letter shapes (Fig. 1, 2). The marking must be located in a non-functional area, for instance outside of the bore contact area or the external polished surface. Machined marking is currently located by manufacturers at the bottom of the ceramic head on an appropriate external chamfer (Fig. 3a). At higher magnification, the size and shape of the grooves can be seen clearly. These grooves are several hundred microns in depth and width (Fig. 1, 2) and must be considered as structural flaws. As a comparison, critical flaws for ceramic materials leading to catastrophic failure are a few tenth microns in size. It is thus critical to avoid any stress concentration in the vicinity of such machined marking. As shown below, this is directly dependent on the location of marking.

(a)   (b)

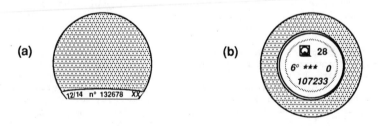

FIG. 3--Schemes of machined marking at the bottom of the head (a) and Laser engraving at the top of the bore (b)

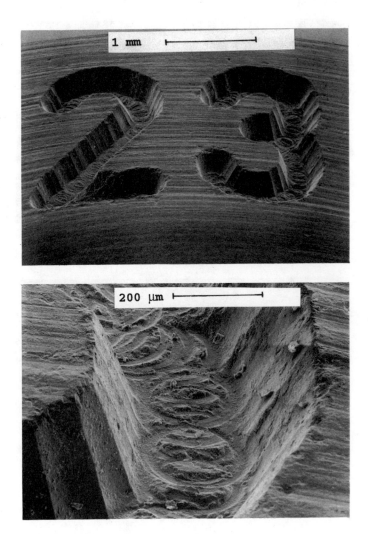

FIG. 1--Microstructure of machined marking using small drills.

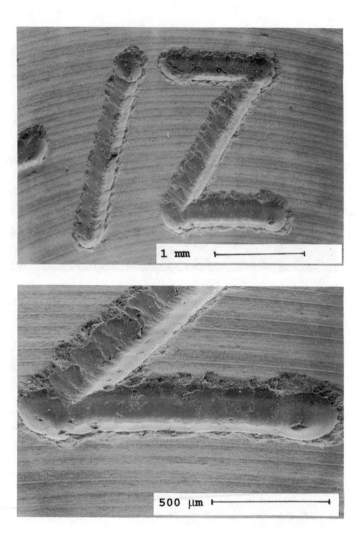

FIG. 2--Microstructure of machined marking using needle-punches.

The use of machined marking could also induce other microstructural flaws due to mechanical stresses generated by the small drills. Small splinters can be observed when very thin shapes are machined. Similarly small chips are observed in the bottom of the grooves (Fig. 4). The size of these secondary flaws is negligible compared to the size of the groove itself.

Mechanical marking done with a needle-punch generates a smooth layer having low adherence with the bulk. However, the edge of the grooves are very rough because of chipping during green marking (Fig. 4). Formation of ceramic debris from this area under mechanical stress could be a problem.

At very high magnification, the microstructure of the material inside the grooves is observed. The surface roughness is quite high and the grains appear smooth because of their thermal etching during sintering.

Laser Beam Marking

Laser beam marking is also used for biomedical products. Marking results from a local melting of the material under the laser beam. Specific difficulties can be observed in using such marking techniques for bioceramics and precise laser marking conditions must be defined. This is due to the high temperatures and thermal shocks associated with the laser beam and to the poor thermal conductivity of oxide ceramics: alumina and zirconia.

In the particular case of zirconia, the engraved material becomes black. This is convenient for a clear legibility of the marked information in so far as zirconia ceramics have normally a white or ivory color. The change in color corresponds to a loss of oxygen that results from the difference in oxygen activity (a_{O2}) between zirconia ceramic ($a_{O2} = 1$) and surrounding atmosphere (air : $a_{O2} \approx 0.32$) during laser marking. Oxygen diffuses from high to low activity area giving a deviation from the stoechiometric composition ZrO_2. However under laser marking conditions, the deviation to stoechiometry is small and probably shall not exceed 10^{-4}, thus corresponding to a final composition $ZrO_{1,9999}$ [9]. This change only concerns the electronic structure of the material and has no influence on its macroscopic mechanical properties, i.e. fracture strength of toughness.

The conditions of laser engraving for ceramic marking must be carefully optimized. If the laser beam is too energetic large melted areas are created at the surface of the material (Fig. 5). The marking shown in Figure 5 has been obtained with an inappropriate pulsed laser technique. The laser beam generated marked holes at the surface. A large volume of melted material was splashed on the surface.

Under controlled and optimized conditions, laser marking leads to a very thin melted layer without cracking zirconia (Fig. 6). At higher magnification, one can see that the ceramic surface is slightly changed by the laser beam (Fig. 6). At the same magnification (x 500), the surface of machined marking appears very rough and microcracked (compare Fig. 4 to 6). The thickness of the melted layer clearly appears on a fractured sample (Fig. 7). Melted material is made of characteristic columnar grains, while bulk material is made of equiaxial grains. Under

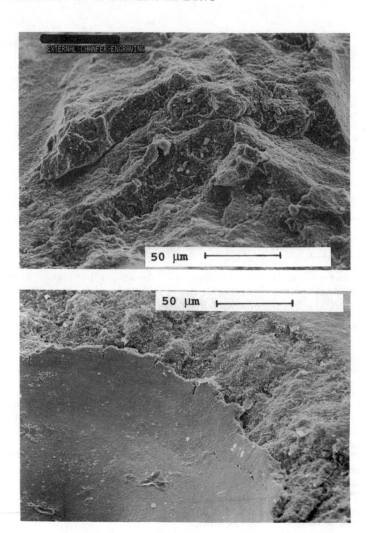

FIG. 4--Microstructure of machined marking using small drills (a) or needle-punches (b) [high magnification]

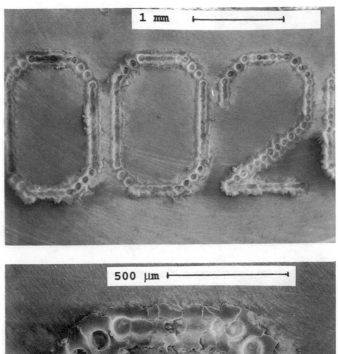

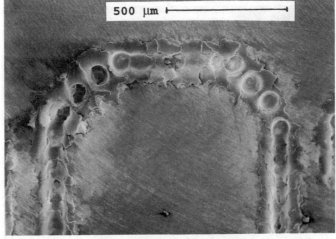

FIG. 5--Microstructure of laser engraved ceramic (inappropriate conditions).

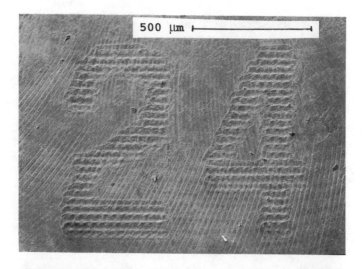

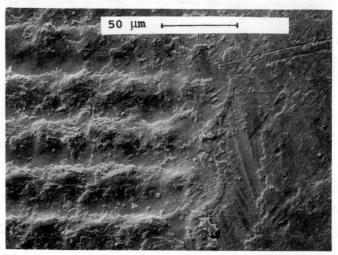

FIG. 6--Microstructure of the Laser engraved ceramic (optimized
conditions).

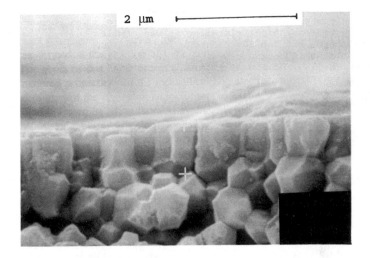

FIG. 7--Laser engraved material (cross section).

optimized conditions, the melted layer is about 1 μm thick. This is
considerably lower than the size of the grooves for machined marking
which are a few hundred microns deep. Optimized laser marking thus leads
to very small flaws, the size of which are significantly smaller than
critical flaws (assumed to be a few tenth microns [10]).

Most of the manufacturers using laser engraving make the marking at
the top of the ceramic bore (Fig. 3b).

MECHANICAL CONSEQUENCE OF MARKING

The influence of laser marking on the fracture strength of a zirconia
bioceramic (PROZYR®) has been measured using the 3 point flexural test on
rectangular bars (4 x 2 x 24 mm). Two "OO" letters were laser engraved in
the middle of the tensile side of the flexural bars. The comparison of
laser engraved and non-engraved test bars indicates that under optimized
conditions, the reduction in strength due to laser marking is lower than
15%. Similarly, an "X" was mechanically engraved on green rectangular
bars before sintering. The shape of engraved labels was chosen for
feasability reasons. After sintering it was similar to that observed in
commercial heads and had 200 μm about in depth. Due to the size of this
groove, a strong reduction (about 45%) in fracture strength was observed.
Table 1 summarizes the flexural strength and standard deviation in both
cases (8 bars were used in each test).

TABLE 1--Comparison of flexural strength change for laser and
mechanically engraved test bars (8 bars per test)

| | Flexural strength (MPa) | | Variation |
| | Non engraved bars | Engraved bars | |
	Mean (Std dev)	Mean (Std dev)	%
Laser engraving	949 (90)	820 (56)	13
Mechanical marking	872 (86)	478 (108)	45

The use of the statistical q (Studentized range) test [11]
confirms, with a significance level of 99%, that the mean fracture
strength of mechanically engraved and non-engraved bars are significantly
different. In the case of laser engraving the significance level is only
≤ 90%, because of the lower flexural strength change.

The influence of laser engraving on mechanical properties has also
been investigated on zirconia femoral heads (PROZYR®). This has been done
on 28 mm zirconia femoral heads [neck length 0, 14/16 taper] using the
ISO 7206-5 standard burst test on Ti-6Al-4V trunnions. The burst strength
of 20 heads, laser-engraved at the top of the bore, were compared to the
burst strength of 20 non-engraved zirconia heads. Marked information
followed the ISO 6018 standard requirements (Fig. 2b) : head diameter,
taper angle, neck length, unitary head number, end-user reference. As
shown in Table 2, the two head populations are characterized by the same
mean fracture strength and standard deviation.

TABLE 2--Comparison of fracture strength of laser engraved and non-engraved femoral heads

	Fracture strength Engraved heads kN	Fracture strength Non-engraved heads kN
Mean Value	124	125
Maximum Value	135	139
Minimum Value	107	107
Standard Deviation	7	11

    The fracture strength of laser engraved and non-engraved zirconia heads are also compared in Figure 8 using a Weibull plot, where the probability of rupture P is plotted versus fracture strength. It is observed that the two head populations are characterized by the same Weibull modulus (slope of the extrapolated line) indicating the same scattering of fracture strength for engraved and non-engraved zirconia femoral heads.

    Therefore, it may be concluded that laser marking of zirconia heads, provided it is made in optimized conditions (marking procedure), does not induce measurable strength degradation.

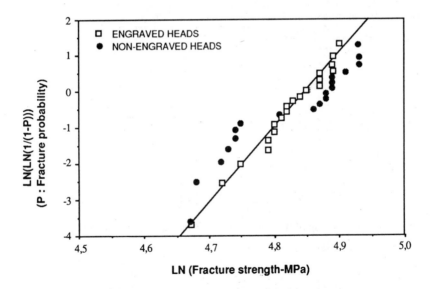

FIG. 8--Fracture strength of engraved and non-engraved 28 mm zirconia femoral heads (Neck length 0 - 14/16 taper)

The influence of mechanical marking on the fracture strength of the same heads could not be evaluated, because non-marked samples were not available.

The location of marking is also of prime importance for the reliability of the femoral heads. Under service, some stress concentrations are generated inside the head, the level of which depends on patient morphology and activity. The location of these stress concentrations must be identified and the marking made outside these areas. For most ceramic head designs, the highest stress concentration is located at the interface between metallic trunnion and ceramic bore [7,8]. However, stress concentrations extend into the bulk and could affect to a lower degree either the top of the ceramic cone or the bottom of the head, or both [7,8]. The stress map must be analyzed for each head design in order to verify that the marking is made in low stress areas.

This will be particularly sensitive for the small ceramic heads, for instance with 22.22mm diameter, the use of which is increasing rapidly. As previously shown [7,8], two main stress concentrations are observed in the head under loading. The first one at the top of the bore is limited to the corner, while the second at the bottom of the head, concern a larger area and may extend up to the external chamfer where machined marking is currently located. The stress profiles in these two regions, deduced from Finite Element Analysis, are plotted in figure 9 versus the path at either the top of the bore or at the outer surface. The stress level is significantly higher at the bottom of the head than at the top of the bore in the areas where the marking is made. In addition, if we consider that the flaws introduced by machined marking are two orders of magnitude larger than that corresponding to laser marking, then laser engraving at the top of the ceramic bore must be a much more conservative marking technique which can guarantee long term reliability.

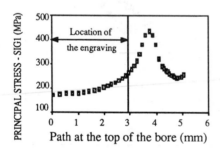

Path at the top of the bore (mm)   Path at the bottom of the head (mm)

FIG. 9--Stress profile at the top of the bore and at the bottom of the head. Head design: Ø 22.22 mm - Long neck - Applied load: 45 kN

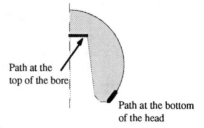

CONCLUSIONS

Marking of ceramic hip joint heads allows good traceability and is required in normal biomedical practice. Two main techniques are used for femoral head marking: machining and laser engraving. Furthermore, two areas on the heads are concerned : the top of the bore and the bottom of the head.

It is observed that:

- the structural flaws associated with ceramic head marking are two orders of magnitude larger for machined marking than for laser engraving,

- the stress concentration at the bottom of the head could be significantly higher than at the top of the bore and concern a larger area.

Since machined marking is preferably made at the bottom of the head while laser engraving is currently performed at the top of the bore, it is argued that laser engraving at the top of the ceramic bore is a more suitable marking procedure to guarantee long term reliability.However, the stress situation must be analyzed for each head design on the basis of the stress map supplied by Finite Element Analysis, especially for marking at the bottom of the head where tensile stresses could be higher.

REFERENCES

[1]   Boutin, P., "Total Arthroplasty of the Hip by Sintered Alumina Prosthesis. Experimental Study and 1st Clinical Applications, " Rev. Chir. Ortop., Vol. 58, 1972, pp 229-246.

[2]   Griss, P. and G. Heimke, "Five Years Experience with Ceramic-Metal-Composite Hip Endoprostheses. I:Clinical Evaluation, " Arch. Orthop. Traumat. Surg., Vol. 98,   1981, pp 157-164.

[3]   Semlitsch, M., Lehmann, M., Weber, H., Doerre, E., and H- G. Willert, "New Prospect for a Prolonged Functional Life-span of Artificial Hip Joint by Using the Material Combination Polyethylene/Aluminium Oxide Ceramic/Metal, " J. Biomed.Mater. Res., Vol. 11, 1977, pp   537-552.

[4]   Zichner, L. P., and Willert, H-G., "Comparison of Alumina-Polyethylene and Metal-Polyethylene in Clinical Trials : Alumina Ceramic Arthroplasty, " Clinical Orthop. Related Res., Vol. 292, 1992, pp 86-94.

[5]   Clarke, I. C., "Role of Ceramic Implants : Design and Clinical Success with Total Hip Prosthetic Ceramic-to-ceramic Bearings : Alumina Ceramic Arthroplasty, " Clinical Orthop. Related Res. , Vol. 282, 1992, pp 19-30.

[6]   Schuller, H. and R. Marti, "Ten-year Socket Wear in 66 Arthroplasties. Ceramic versus Metal Heads, " Acta Orthop. Scand. , Vol. 61, 1990, pp 240-243.

[7]   Drouin, J.M. and B. Calès, "Finite Element Analysis of Stress in Zirconia Femoral Heads, " Actualités en Biomatériaux, Editions Romillat, Paris, 1993.

[8]. Drouin, J.M. and B. Calès, "Yttria-Stabilized Zirconia Ceramic for Improved Hip Joint Head, " <u>Bioceramics - Vol. 7</u>, Butterworth-Heinemann, London, 1994.

[9]   Olette, M. and M.F. Ancey-Moret, "Variation of Free Energy of Formation of Oxides and Nitrides with Temperature, "<u>Revue de Metallurgie</u> ,June 1963, pp 569-580.

[10] Kingery, W. D. , Bowen, H. K. and Uhlmann, D. R., "<u>Introduction to Ceramics, 2nd Editon</u> , " pp 769-815, John Wiley & Sons Publishers, New York , 1976.

[11] Lang-Michaut, C., "<u>Practice of statistical tests- Analysis of measurements,</u> " Ed. Bordas,Paris(1990).

State of the Art in Properties Testing I

Mary E. Anthony[1], Michael B. Cooper[1], and Jeffrey A. Holbrook[1]

TEST METHOD FOR FATIGUE OF A MODULAR POSTERIOR-STABILIZED TIBIAL COMPONENT

REFERENCE: Anthony, M. E., Cooper, M. B., and Holbrook, J. A., "**Test Method for Fatigue of a Modular Posterior-Stabilized Tibial Component,**" *Modularity of Orthopedic Implants, ASTM STP 1301,* Donald E. Marlowe, Jack E. Parr, and Michael B. Mayor, Eds., American Society for Testing and Materials, 1997.

ABSTRACT: Posterior-stabilized (P/S) total knee replacements are designed to replace the function of the knee joint in the absence of the posterior cruciate ligament. The most prevalent P/S tibial components are modular, consisting of a plastic tibial insert which is secured by the locking mechanism to a metallic tibial tray. While these tibial components offer the advantages of modularity including increased flexibility and decreased inventory, they must withstand loading that will be transferred to the tibial insert post, without excessive deformation of the post or disassociation of the tibial insert from the tibial tray. The objective of this study is to develop a test method to determine the fatigue integrity of a modular P/S tibial component under physiologic loading.

Modular P/S tibial components are subjected to a combined compressive and anteroposterior shear load transferred from the femoral component to the tibial insert post and the condylar surfaces. A test method was developed to reproduce this loading by placing a P/S implant at 30° of flexion and transferring load to the tibial component as would occur in vivo. By applying a 5 Hz, sinusoidal load in this manner for ten million cycles, the fatigue integrity of the modular component can be evaluated. Additional information may be gained by measuring the angular deformation of the tibial insert post and determining the static locking strength of the tibial construct after fatigue loading. Failure criteria for the modular component would be either disassociation of the tibial insert or gross deformation of the tibial insert post.

KEYWORDS: total knee arthroplasty, posterior-stabilized total knee arthroplasty

[1]Research Engineers and Senior Research Technician, respectively. Technical Services Department, Smith & Nephew Richards Inc., 1450 Brooks Rd., Memphis, TN 38116, USA.

BACKGROUND

Posterior-stabilized (P/S) knee prostheses consisting of a P/S femoral component and a modular tibial component are commonly used in total knee replacement surgeries. The tibial component includes an ultrahigh molecular weight polyethylene (UHMWPE) tibial insert with a post and a metallic tibial tray. The P/S design is unique from a cruciate retaining design, having an additional structural metallic box and/or cam on the interior surface of the femoral component and an UHMWPE post on the modular tibial insert. The design of the P/S option is such that the cam on the femoral component contacts the post on the tibial insert. This mechanism prevents dislocation of the femoral component anteriorly and replaces the function that the posterior cruciate ligament would perform in a normal knee.

Clinical failures of modular P/S tibial components may result from disassociation of the tibial insert, dislocation of the femoral component, and/or loss of structural integrity of the tibial insert post [1, 2]. Testing of a modular P/S tibial component should be performed to ensure that the integrity of the tibial locking mechanism and tibial insert post are sufficient to withstand in vivo loading. An optimal test method would transfer the same magnitudes and types of loading to the component as are expected clinically. The ability of the tibial component to survive such loading would serve as one safety indicator for the success of the modular design.

OBJECTIVE

The purpose of this test method is to ensure the fatigue integrity of a modular P/S tibial component under worst case physiologic loading. The modular tibial component will be loaded by way of the appropriate femoral component, as would occur in vivo. At the completion of fatigue testing, both the tibial locking strength and the amount of tibial insert post deformation will be determined. The resulting data can be used to evaluate the design of a modular P/S tibial component.

PARAMETERS

As loading at the knee joint is significant, and includes frequent repetition such as in level walking, the integrity of the modular tibial component should be evaluated in fatigue. The type of loading, the loading angle, the applied load, and the component size should mimic expected worst case clinical conditions.

Type of Loading

As the knee begins to flex, the femoral condyles roll back on the tibia. As flexion continues, sliding of the femur anteriorly occurs simultaneous to rolling. At high angles of flexion, sliding alone occurs. This motion results in loading at the knee joint which is a combination of compression, shear, and torsion. During sliding, the bar on the P/S femoral implant applies a load to the tibial insert post a given distance from the locking mechanism, resulting in an additional bending moment. Important to the evaluation of the design of a modular P/S tibial component are the compressive force, which works to hold the components together and resist dislocation, and the anteroposterior shear force, which requires the function of the femoral stabilizing bar and tibial insert post to resist dislocation. The bending moment that occurs within the implant must also be accounted for. To reproduce this loading, this test method places the components at a specified angle of flexion. In flexion, a compressive and an anteroposterior shear load result in an applied bending moment tending to remove the insert from the tibial tray or to deform/fracture the tibial insert post.

Loading Angle

It is important to evaluate the position of the knee in flexion where maximum compressive and anteroposterior loads occur. By overlaying the work of Seireg and Arvikar [3] and Murray et al [4] (Figure 1), it is evident that maximum anteroposterior loads in the knee occur at about 50-55% of the walking cycle, or about 15-25° of flexion [3, 4]. At these low angles of flexion, the bar of the femoral component generally would not contact the tibial insert post. A more pertinent loading peak in the anteroposterior direction occurs at about 55-60% of the walking cycle [3], which correlates to about 30-40° of flexion [4]. As the bar of the femoral component could potentially load the tibial insert post at 30° of flexion, this position is chosen for testing. Anteroposterior loads that occur at higher angles of flexion are lesser in magnitude [3] and would occur at a more inferior position on the post. Superior loading of the post increases the distance from the point of load application to the tray locking mechanism and therefore increases the moment tending to disengage the tibial insert from the tibial tray. Loading the post at 30° of flexion, therefore, represents a worst case physiologic condition.

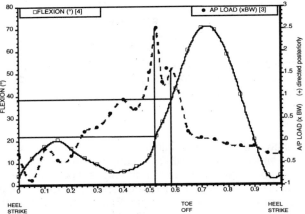

FIG. 1--Angle of Flexion and Anteroposterior Shear Force in the Knee During Level Walking

Applied Load

The load applied to the P/S construct should be representative of that predicted in vivo. Based on studies by Seireg and Arvikar, Paul, and Morrison, the maximum resultant load predicted at the knee joint during level walking ranges from 3.0-7.1 times body weight (BW) [3, 5, 6]. Seireg and Arvikar further defined the anteroposterior component of this load to be a maximum of 2.5 x BW with a second peak at 1.8 x BW [3]. Therefore, one possible simulation of in vivo loading would include a compressive component of approximately 5 x BW and an anteroposterior shear component of approximately 2 x BW.

If testing is performed at 30° of flexion, then an applied load would result in the following force components:

$$Fc = Fr * \cos (\emptyset) \qquad (1)$$
$$Fap = Fr * \sin (\emptyset) \qquad (2)$$

where

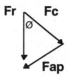

Fc = Compressive Force Component
Fr = Resultant Force = Applied Load
∅   = Flexion Angle
Fap = Anteroposterior Force Component

If a 1000 lbf. (4450 N) load is chosen for application to the assembly at 30° of flexion, the resulting force components would be:

Fc = 866 lbf. (3854 N)
Fap = 500 lbf. (2225 N)

Assuming a body weight of 167 lbf. (743 N):

Fc = 5.2 x BW
Fap = 3.0 x BW

Thus a resultant applied load of 1000 lbf. (4450 N) would subject the assembly to one combination of compressive and anteroposterior loading as predicted during in vivo use.

Component Size

The presence of a modular P/S tibial insert allows for various tibial thicknesses as well as sizes. As with any test protocol, it is important to evaluate the size and thickness that would result in the highest potential for failure. In this test, the thickest size tibial component offered should be used to ensure that the bending moment produced is at a maximum (Figure 2). The size of the components to be tested should be such that they result in the greatest possibility for lock disassociation. For most designs, the smallest components would contain the smallest locking area and would thus be worst case. However, each design should be evaluated to determine the most severe test case.

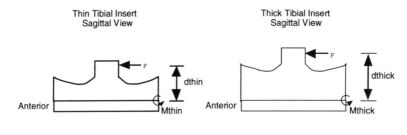

FIG. 2--The Effect of Tibial Component Thickness

METHODS

The modular P/S tibial component must withstand predicted in vivo loading transferred to the tibial insert post without disengagement of the modular connection. Also, the P/S UHMWPE tibial insert post must resist excessive deformation and/or fracture under load.

The fatigue integrity of the construct, the amount of post deformation, and the static strength of the locking mechanism measured after fatigue loading would be of interest in determining the long term performance of the design.

Fatigue Test Parameters

A P/S tibial insert shall be placed in a tibial tray which is fixed in a potting medium (for example, polymethylmethacrylate). The tibial insert/tibial tray assembly will then be secured to the moving actuator of the test machine at 30° of flexion. A P/S femoral component shall be attached to the load cell mounted at the top of the test machine such that the tibial insert post is loaded via the bar on the posterior side of the P/S femoral component (Figure 3). A 5 Hz, sinusoidal load of 100/1000 lbf. (445/4450 N) will be applied to the assembly until failure or until completion of ten million cycles of loading. Failure will be defined as disassociation of the tibial insert from the tibial tray or excessive deformation of the tibial insert post such that it can no longer withstand applied loading.

Post Deformation

The amount of deformation of the tibial insert post in the posterior to anterior direction should be measured for all constructs completing ten million loading cycles without failure. An outline of the tibial insert post can be made on an optical comparator prior to each test; this outline can then be compared to that taken post-fatigue. The amount of angular deformation due to the fatigue loading can then be measured and recorded. The amount of deformation can provide information as to the ability of the tibial insert post to maintain its integrity when subjected to worst case loading.

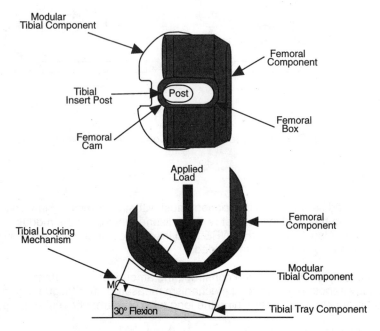

FIG. 3--Schematic of the Fatigue Test Setup

<u>Post-Fatigue Locking Strength</u>

Static locking strength of the modular, P/S construct can be measured for all constructs that complete ten million loading cycles without failure. This strength can be compared to the static locking strength of previously untested components to determine if the integrity of the locking mechanism has been affected. For this test, components will be placed at 30° of flexion and load will be applied to the tibial insert post via the bar on the femoral component at a rate of 0.1 in. /min. (0.042 mm/sec.). Testing will continue until the insert dislocates from the tibial tray. Load versus deflection should be recorded.

AREAS TO ADDRESS

This test method attempts to determine the integrity of a modular P/S tibial component under expected in vivo loading. The test method allows for physiologic loading to be applied to the construct, and evaluates the resulting performance of the design. However, several problems with this test method should be addressed. These include limiting the testing to one angle of flexion, heating of the polyethylene tibial insert, stiffness of the test setup, and repeatability of the results.

Single Angle of Flexion

This test method is performed with the P/S knee components placed at 30° of flexion. While this angle of flexion simulates what is seen clinically, and results in a combined compressive and anteroposterior load of the magnitude expected in vivo, it remains a simplification of actual motion of the knee during level walking. Realistically, during walking, the knee is flexed from about 5-70° [4]. As the knee is flexed, loading of the joint and prosthesis changes. By limiting the testing to 30° of flexion, a worst case loading is applied, but the situation is magnified. For a more realistic simulation of loading and motion patterns, a multi-axis joint simulator would be required. In the absence of this expensive, elaborate equipment, this test method still produces a simulation of the clinical situation.

Heating of the Polyethylene

The knee is not continuously cycled in vivo; in fact it receives frequent rest periods. In this test, the loading is continually applied. Also, in this test, the frequency of motion, 5 Hz, exceeds that of a typical walking pattern (approximately 1 Hz). Lastly, this test is performed in air, and thus no fluid is allowed into the joint surfaces. The result is that the UHMWPE may be subject to excessive heating which could lead to premature failure. In order to compensate for this problem, a small flow of air can be directed toward the tibial insert during testing. This allows completion of the test in a timely manner without unexpected results. An alternative method would be to perform this testing in a fluid bath and/or occasionally stop the test to allow for cooling of the UHMWPE tibial insert.

Stiffness of the Test Setup

Considerable bending results from the proposed test setup. The fixturing for the test must be of sufficient stiffness to ensure that the load is transmitted to the assembly and not taken up by the fixturing.

Repeatability

Setup of the test is critical to producing accurate, reproducible results. It is imperative that the assembly be configured such that the load is evenly distributed on the medial and lateral condyles. Verification of this criteria can be obtained by placing contact film in the condylar surfaces. Also, it is important that the bar on the P/S femoral component is placed such that it contacts the tibial insert post in a consistent manner. Again, verification with contact paper is recommended. A method for ensuring the exact load transferred to the condylar surfaces and tibial insert post would also be beneficial.

ADDITIONAL APPLICATIONS

In addition to the evaluation of modular P/S tibial designs, this test method could also be modified to allow analysis of similar components. Monolithic, all-UHMWPE P/S tibial components are now used in total knee replacement surgery. Though the modular interface is no longer present in these designs, the tibial insert post must still resist similar loading without excessive deformation or fracture. Also, the strength of the tibial component/cement layer is important to ensure that loosening of the implant does not occur.

A second application involves the increased trend toward conforming, anterior-lipped tibial inserts for cruciate retaining total knee replacements. Though these tibial inserts are indicated for use in patients with a functioning posterior cruciate ligament, they must still resist dislocation from the metal backing. If the femoral component loads the anterior edge of the implant, there is a bending moment applied which would tend to dislocate the tibial insert (Figure 4). Therefore, this test method could be modified to load the anterior edge of the tibial insert.

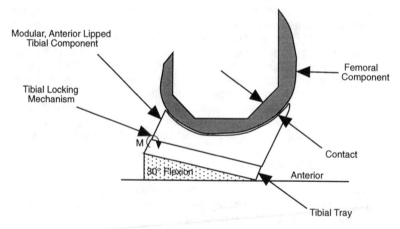

FIG. 4--Testing of a Modular, Anterior Lipped Tibial Component

CONCLUSIONS

In conclusion, a test method is presented which determines the fatigue integrity of a modular P/S tibial component under physiologic loading. The method involves subjecting the P/S femoral and tibial assembly to a combined compressive and anteroposterior shear load transferred from the femoral component to the tibial insert post and the condylar surfaces. The test evaluates potential failure modes including: dislocation of the tibial insert and excessive deformation or fracture of the tibial insert post such that it can no longer withstand expected loading.

REFERENCES

[1] Lumbardi, A. V., et al, "Dislocation Following Primary Posterior-Stabilized Total Knee Arthroplasty," Journal of Arthroplasty, Vol. 8, No. 6, 1993, pp. 633-639.

[2] Striplin, D. B. And Robinson, R. P., "Posterior Dislocation of the Insall /Burstein II Posterior Stabilized Total Knee Prosthesis," The American Journal of Knee Surgery, Vol. 5, No. 2, Spring 1992, pp. 79-83.

[3] Seireg, A. and Arvikar, R. J., "The Prediction of Muscular Load Sharing and Joint Forces in the Lower Extremities During Walking," Journal of Biomechanics, Vol. 8, 1975, pp. 89-102.

[4] Murray, et al, "Walking Patterns of Normal Men," Journal of Bone and Joint Surgery, Vol. 64-A, No. 2, March 1964, pp. 335-360.

[5] Paul, J. P., "Forces Transmitted by Joints in the Human Body," Proceedings of the Institute of Mechanical Engineers, Vol. 181 Pt. 3J, 1966-67, pp. 8-15.

[6] Morrison, J. B., "The Mechanics of the Knee Joint in Relation to Normal Walking," Journal of Biomechanics, Vol. 3, 1970, pp. 51-61.

Lynn A. Kirkpatrick[1]

TEST METHOD FOR EVALUATING MOTION BETWEEN THE POLYMERIC
ARTICULATING SURFACE AND THE TIBIAL TRAY OF MODULAR TOTAL
KNEE SYSTEMS

REFERENCE: Kirkpatrick, L. A., "**Test Method for Evaluating Motion Between the Polymeric Articulating Surface and the Tibial Tray of Modular Total Knee Systems,**" *Modularity of Orthopedic Implants, ASTM STP 1301,* Donald E. Marlowe, Jack E. Parr, and Michael B. Mayor, Eds., American Society for Testing and Materials, 1997.

ABSTRACT: Anatomic loads that are exerted on the tibial component can result in forces which exert compressive, tensile, and shear stresses in the modular connection between the articular surface and the tibial tray. Stability, as well as strength of the connection, are important to the long-term function of the implant. Consequently, new modular knee designs should be subjected to rigorous analysis and testing to evaluate the modular connection stability.

Component tolerances and locking mechanism design are important to the stability of the interlock. Stability of the interlock is important when evaluating the ability of the design to limit relative motion and the generation of material debris. A static testing technique has been utilized to quantify the amount of relative motion that may occur between the articulating surface and the tibial tray. The method applies a transverse load to the locking mechanism in the plane of the articular surface/tibial tray interface while relative displacement versus load information is collected. With sufficiently low forces, multiple loadings may be applied to the same components for statistical analysis. Tests with displacements ranging from 0.13 to 0.56 mm have shown standard deviation ranges of 0.6 percent to 8.6 percent.

A plot of the force versus displacement data is useful in the analysis of the locking mechanism performance. Regions of movement, or sliding, between the components are indicated by a relatively low slope in the curve. A relatively high slope will indicate regions of stiffness of the mechanism. The results may then be used to compare the performance of the specimens with clinically successful designs.

KEYWORDS: total knee, modular, tibial tray

---

[1]Senior Research Engineer, Biomechanical Testing, Zimmer, Inc., P.O. Box 708, Warsaw, IN 46581-0708

INTRODUCTION

The articular surface-to-tibial tray locking mechanism of the modular tibial components in a total knee prosthesis serve two primary functions: to maintain assembly of the components, and to limit relative motion between the articular surface and tibial tray. Relative motion has the potential to contribute wear debris to the joint system. Many factors play a role in determining the effectiveness of the locking mechanism to limit relative component motion, including geometry, tolerances, and material properties.

A method has been developed to measure the relative motion (or sliding) that may occur between the Ultra-High Molecular-Weight Polyethylene (UHMWPE) articular surface (AS) and the tibial tray (TT) of a modular tibial component resulting from loads applied parallel to and in the plane of contact of the components. The motion is measured in the plane of contact of the components in the medial-lateral and anterior-posterior directions. No compressive (joint load) is applied during this test. This procedure is used as a tool to compare the relative motion between designs, or design iterations.

To perform the experiment, a universal tensile tester has been used, but a servo-hydraulic loadframe may also be employed (Fig. 1). With appropriate fixtures, the TT and AS were assembled and mounted in a loadframe which was capable of applying controlled displacement. During the experiment the loadframe/data acquisition system must be capable of accurately recording force and displacement. A strain-gauge extensometer was used to record displacements in order to achieve the appropriate level of displacement measurement accuracy, 0.0025 mm. The extensometer was mounted to a spring loaded follower which was positioned against the components.

In this method a transverse force is applied to the AS while the TT is held stationary. The force is applied parallel to the transverse plane of contact between the AS and TT components. A force applied in a direction other than parallel to the interface plane would apply either a compressive or distractive force component to the locking mechanism and could be a source of bias in the results.

This procedure is intended to be used only for comparison purposes. It is not considered to be a simulation of *in vivo* function nor is it considered to be an evaluation of TT-to-AS interface strength. Interface strength can be determined by other methods, depending upon the family, or type of implant and the anticipated loading.

MATERIALS AND METHODS

This test can be performed in a universal tensile tester or a suitable device which can record load versus displacement. A crosshead displacement speed of 0.254 mm per minute has been used.

The TT is rigidly connected to the tester with a fixture block by one of two methods. Screws are used through fixation holes if screws are used for *in vivo* component

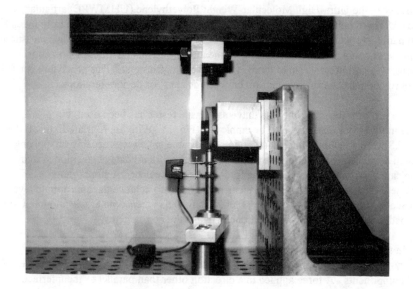

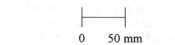

0   50 mm

FIG. 1--Test setup.

fixation. If the design relies on bone cement or other means of fixation, structural adhesive (i.e., Scotchweld 2214 from Adhesives, Coatings and Selaers Division, St. Paul, MN, or Torr Seal from Varian Associates, Vacuum Division, Palo Alto, CA) is used. The mounting surface of the fixture block must conform to and support the TT underside to prevent distortion of the AS contact surface which may affect the results (Fig. 2). Clearance may be provided for stems or projections on the TT underside in lieu of removing them.

The AS is connected to a separate fixture plate which is attached to the tester force transducer. It is critical that the attachment method does not distort the AS, thus influencing the fit between the components. This has been accomplished by drilling a hole through each condylar surface. The hole is countersunk on the underside for a flathead screw. Spherical washers or special spacers are placed between the transducer fixture plate and articulation face of the AS to facilitate the parallel alignment of the AS with respect to the TT. Flathead screws are inserted through from the AS underside, through the washers, and tightened into the fixture plate (Fig. 3). The use of flathead screws provides a low profile while the conical shape seats in the conical countersinks to eliminate the possible influence of any clearance between the screw shank and holes in the AS. Care must be taken not to over-torque the screws. With thin and/or small components it may be possible to expand the AS, thus influencing component fit. Component dimensions may be checked before and after the screws are torqued to verify that no expansion has occurred during tightening. The amount of offset, or lateral distance from the AS/TT contact plane to the transducer fixture plate should be minimized to reduce deflection or nonparallelism that may result during testing.

The TT and mounting fixture assembly is attached to the crosshead of the tester. When in position, but not assembled, parallelism between components is checked. The run out of each component with respect to the other is measured while moving the tester crosshead. Shims and adjusting screws are used, as required, to reduce nonparallelism between the components. With relatively small displacements (less than 0.5 mm), a total nonparallelism of 5 degrees is acceptable, depending on the design of the locking mechanism. Excessive nonparallelism will result in compressive or distractive forces which may bias test results. The components are then assembled and positioned in the tester using the fixturing required to maintain parallelism.

A strain-gauge extensometer has been used for displacement measurements. The extensometer is mounted on a spring-loaded follower that is secured to the same base as one of the component fixtures, typically the TT (Fig. 4). With the extensometer follower contacting the other component, typically the AS, relative movement between the component specimens can be accurately measured when the tester crosshead is moved. Alternative devices, such as LVDT's or lasers, may be used to measure displacement if they have sufficient accuracy.

To determine how much of measured movement is truly AS-to-TT looseness, compliance of the stationary component and the fixture is also measured. This is done by

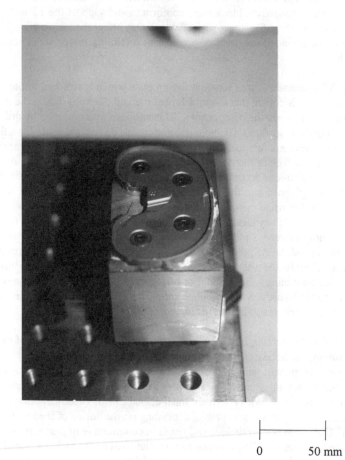

0   50 mm

FIG. 2--Tibial tray attached to test fixture.

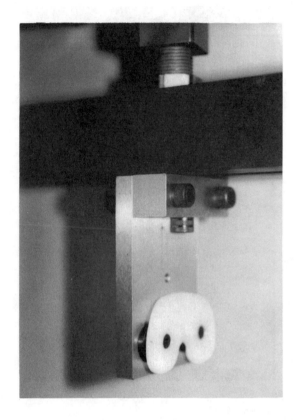

0   50 mm

FIG. 3--Articular surface attached to test fixture.

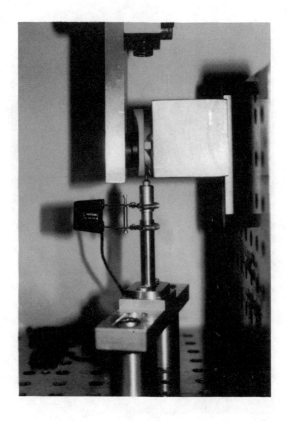

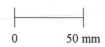

0   50 mm

FIG. 4--Extensometer contacting articular surface.

repositioning the extensometer and plunger to contact the TT. The crosshead is moved and any TT movement due to fixture compliance is measured. The difference of the two measurements, TT and AS, is the actual AS-to-TT movement.

The test is conducted by applying the force from a relative "negative" to "positive" sense upon the components with the moving of the tester crosshead. The relative motion of the components is measured in a single movement, or excursion of the tester during the run. An initial, "negative" force is applied by manually moving the crosshead until the desired force is applied to the assembled specimens. Values of +/-222N have been used for the positive and negative forces. However, the magnitude used may be dependent on the locking mechanism design. The tester crosshead is started in the opposite direction, moving the AS component in a single movement of the tester crosshead until the desired "positive" force has been attained. Displacements are recorded at the desired force magnitudes and force displacement curves are generated.

Performance of the locking mechanism can be determined in both the M-L and A-P directions by positioning the components in the appropriate orientations in the tester.

RESULTS AND DISCUSSION

This procedure has evolved through several iterations to the form described in this paper. In using the described procedure, standard deviations of 0.6 percent to 8.6 percent have been obtained for specimens with total displacements ranging from 0.13 to 0.56 mm.

Serig and Arvikar [1] found A-P joint forces to range from approximately -2.2 to +1.0 times bodyweight. They also found M-L forces to range from -1.0 to +0.8 times bodyweight. The forces currently used in this method are +/-222 N (50 pounds) for both the M-L and A-P directions. Initially, anatomic load forces were attempted in this method. However, at the higher loads it was difficult to maintain parallelism between the components due to component and fixture deflection. The use of the lower force magnitude allows multiple runs of the test for each assembly for statistical analysis, while reducing the possibility of damaging locking mechanism. If deformation of the components is suspected, or occurs, it can be detected by close inspection of the force versus displacement curves. A shifting, or progressive change in the curves indicates the components have been affected.

This procedure will yield relative values of modular component motion. By examining the slope, or changing slope of the force-displacement curves, areas of motion and areas of stiffness can be seen (Fig. 5). High slope will indicate stiffness of the locking mechanism. The area of the curve with a relatively low slope, signifying movement with small change in force, will indicate low stiffness of the locking mechanism. As the curve slope approaches zero, free "play" may be evident if the assembly was held in the hand and a transverse force applied.

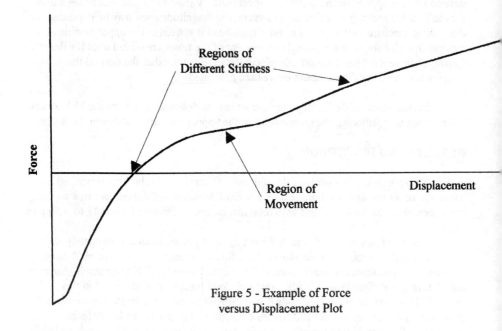

Figure 5 - Example of Force
versus Displacement Plot

It is advisable not to perform the test by applying the force from zero-to-plus and then from zero-to-minus (or visa versa) in separate runs. Significant errors can be introduced when attempting to return to the zero point. If "zero" force is the reference starting point, the position may not be the "zero" displacement point due to looseness. And conversely, if "zero" displacement is the reference starting point, the force may not be the "zero" force point due to looseness. In either case the actual motion is uncertain. By applying the force from minus-to-plus (or visa versa) the shifting "zero" reference point is eliminated.

The use of an extensometer (or lvdt) is strongly advised. The crosshead displacement readouts of even the state-of-the-art universal tensile testers cannot correct for load frame compliance. With the fixtures attached to the components, assembly may be difficult. Allowances must be made in the fixtures which will allow assembly while not damaging the components.

CONCLUSIONS

This procedure is intended only for comparison of the movement of the articular surface with respect to the tibial tray in the plane of contact between the components. Although the preparation and setup require significant amounts of time, the results have been found to be repeatable for given component designs and sizes.

This method is not to be considered an *in vivo* simulation nor can estimates of wear determined. Other test methods must be employed to evaluate the static and fatigue performance of the locking mechanism.

REFERENCE

[1]   A. Serig, R. J. Arvikar, "The Prediction of Muscular Load Sharing and Joint Forces in the Lower Extremities During Walking," J. of Biomechanics, 1075, Vol. 8, pp. 89-102.

Terry W. McLean[1] and Richard D. Lambert[2]

TEST METHOD FOR THE ASSESSMENT OF FRETTING AT THE FEMORAL HEAD AND NECK TAPER INTERFACE

REFERENCE: McLean, T. W. and Lambert, R. D., "Test Method for the Assessment of Fretting at the Femoral Head and Neck Taper Interface," *Modularity of Orthopedic Implants, ASTM STP 1301,* Donald E. Marlowe, Jack E. Parr, and Michael B. Mayor, Eds., American Society for Testing and Materials, 1997.

ABSTRACT: Today in the United States, 95% of all total hip implants contain at least one modular junction. The most common of these junctions connects the femoral head and neck taper. Because this connection utilizes a Morse taper, various materials and design variables can influence fretting and corrosion behavior at the mating surfaces, and ultimately the longevity of the device.

In order to isolate and study the behavior of the femoral head/neck taper connection, a simplified model of a neck taper was designed. Test specimens were manufactured of Ti-6Al-4V and Co-Cr, and were designed to accept a Co-Cr femoral head. These constructs provided control in the experiment by focusing on the femoral head/neck taper interface, and by facilitating debris collection. Each construct was encapsulated with Ringer's solution and subjected to a fatigue load of 490 N to 4900 N at a rate of 10 hertz for ten million cycles. Using direct current plasma-optical emission spectroscopy (DCP-OES), the Ringer's solution was analyzed for titanium and cobalt ions after the fatigue test. The titanium level measured for the Ti-6Al-4V/Co-Cr constructs was less than 0.05 mg/L. For the Ti-6Al-4V/Co-Cr and Co-Cr/Co-Cr constructs, the cobalt levels were 0.95 ± 0.23 mg/L and 1.16 ± 0.57 mg/L, respectively.

This test method was designed to determine the debris generated at the femoral head/neck taper interface by controlling for specific design/fixation variables. It can be used to predict how such factors as material, taper diameter, taper angle, taper

[1] Sr. Research Technician, Device Testing Technical Services, Smith & Nephew Orthopaedics, 1450 Brooks Road, Memphis Tennesses 38116

[2] Sr. Research Engineer, Device Testing Technical Services, Smith & Nephew Orthopaedics, 1450 Brooks Road, Memphis Tennessee 38116

engagement, and tolerances affect the generation of wear debris during fatigue. Although the results do not predict the debris generation of an actual hip prosthesis, they may indicate performance characteristics which can be generalized to in-vivo behavior of the device.

KEYWORDS: fretting, corrosion, modular hip, Morse taper, cobalt, titanium

INTRODUCTION

Modular femoral heads were introduced in the United States in the 1970's [1]. The preferred method of fixation between the head and stem is by means of a friction fit generally referred to as a Morse taper connection. The modular head has gained wide acceptance and gives the surgeon the ability to utilize various materials to optimize the performance of the implant. The surgeon also has the option to adjust the neck length and offset intraoperatively as needed.

There are distinct clinical issues that emerge with any application of a modular device, including fretting, particulate debris, corrosion, and disassociation. A primary concern is the release of metallic particles into the body, inducing an osteolytic response which could result in loosening of the implant. The modular head/neck taper interface has been identified as a contributing source of metallic debris produced in total hip replacement. This debris can be generated mechanically through fretting or chemically by means of corrosion or it may be a combination of both. Fretting can be described as the relative motion between two opposing surfaces which results in the mechanical degradation of one or both surfaces. There are as many opinions as to the types of corrosion that occur at the head/neck taper connection, as there are modular prostheses on the market. Many retrieved components have been noted to exhibit some type of corrosion behavior. Collier attributed the extensive loss of metal to galvanic corrosion on mixed metal head/neck taper connections (Co-Cr/Ti) and not on similar metal connections (Co-Cr/Co-Cr) [2]. All of the mixed metals implants used in this study, however, were produced by the same manufacturer and the mechanical design was not taken into consideration. In recent studies, it appears that better designed and manufactured morse taper connections perform well in-vivo.[3, 4, 5, 6].

OBJECTIVE

The purpose of this study is to develop a test method that will help identify and characterize the wear debris generation at the femoral head/neck taper interface, while controlling specific design/fixation variables.

MATERIALS AND METHODS

This test method provides a way to evaluate the influence of various design variables on the head/neck taper interface as they relate to wear debris generation by using simple neck/taper models. It also allows the head/neck taper interface to be quarantined from any foreign contamination throughout the duration of the test. The isolation of this connection is accomplished through the use of a plastic tube that slides over the test specimen and the femoral head encapsulating the head/neck taper interface as shown in Figure 1.

Five neck taper specimens were manufactured from cobalt-chromium alloy (Co-Cr) and five from Ti-6Al-4V alloy. Each specimen was 76.2 mm in length with a taper diameter of 14.33 mm. A 28 mm diameter Co-Cr head with a +8 mm neck length was chosen as the mating component for these tests. The plastic tube that was used for isolating the head/neck taper connection was 31.75 mm O.D. X 25.4 mm I.D. X 44.5 mm in length.

Preparation of Test Specimens

All components, glassware, and syringes were cleaned individually in a 4% mixture of Micro (International Products Corporation, Burlington, NJ) and ultrapure double deionized water (DDI). The components were placed in an ultrasonic bath and agitated for fifteen minutes at 50°C. They were then rinsed thoroughly using DDI and allowed to air dry for four hours.

Assembly of Test Components

Once dry, each component was hand assembled by placing the head onto the tapered neck specimen. The components were then placed on a servo-hydraulic fatigue frame and an axial compressive load was applied at a rate of 2.54 mm/min. until 2000 N was achieved. The components were then held at that load for one minute, allowing the head to fully seat. The plastic tubing was applied by sliding the tube up from underneath the assembled construct until it almost touched the femoral head. Using DDI, the inside of the construct was then rinsed to remove any plastic shavings or metal particles that could have been generated by assembly of the component. The tubing was then pushed upward until the major diameter of the femoral head was encapsulated. A silicone sealant was used to seal the femoral head and plastic tube interface. The test specimen was then sealed by placing a hose clamp around the base of the tapered neck specimen and plastic tubing. The components were left undisturbed for twelve hours, allowing the sealant to completely cure.

Fixturing of the Assembled Component

Prior to the fixation of the construct to the fatigue frame, 6.0 cc's lactated Ringer's solution (McGraw Inc., Irvine, CA) was injected into the airspace of the plastic tubing with a cleaned syringe.

All of the test specimens were mounted to the fatigue frame at an angle that would allow the load to be applied at 39° to the neck taper axis; this corresponds to loading applied at a 10° angle from the distal stem axis for a femoral stem having a stem/neck angle of 49°. The 10° added laterally is based on ISO standard 7206-3 [7].

Fatigue

A servo-hydraulic fatigue frame was used to load each component from 490 N to 4900 N at a rate of 10 Hz for 10 million cycles. The axial load was transferred through the femoral head via an acetyl resin disc attached to a bearing plate. The applied load was approximately six times body weight which has been measured in previous studies under various activities[8,9]. A schematic of the test set-up is shown in Figure 1.

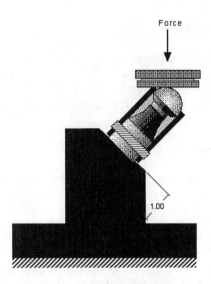

Fig. 1--Schematic of Test Set-up

Solution Extraction, Preparation, and Analysis

After completion of ten million cycles, the testing solution was extracted from the component using a clean syringe, and placed in a 60 cc plastic Nalgene container. In order to remove as much debris as possible, 6.0 cc's of DDI was then injected into the airspace of the tubing and agitated for two minutes using an ultrasonic cleaner. The DDI was then extracted and added to the original Ringer's test solution to make up the master solution. The volume of the master solution was then diluted to a total of 50 cc's to ensure enough solution for ion analysis.

One cubic centimeter of hydrofluoric (HF) and hydrochloric (HCL) acid at a ratio 1:1 was added to 25 cc's of the master solution to dissolve all the metal particles into ionic form. The sample was then sent to Teledyne Wah Chang Albany (Albany, OR) for ion analysis using direct current plasma-optical emission spectroscopy (DCP-OES). Co and Ti ions were measured for each of the ten tests.

Femoral Head Disengagement

After the solution had been extracted, the plastic tubing that encapsulated the femoral head/neck taper interface was removed and the specimen was allowed to dry. Each of the femoral head/neck taper specimens was then secured to an MTS 810 System (MTS Systems Corporation, Eden Prairie, MN) and the femoral head was disengaged from the neck taper specimen at a rate of 2.54 mm/min. The maximum disengagement force was measured and recorded on an X-Y plotter.

RESULTS

Disengagement

The average disengagement force for the five similar and five mixed metal test components was approximately 4307 ± 1055 N and 3612 ± 1015 N, respectively.

Visual Inspection of the Tapers

After disengagement, the contact area of the tapered neck specimens and femoral heads was visually inspected for surface damage. The Co-Cr tapered neck specimens revealed little to no noticeable damage on the contact surface area. Damage was not observed on the contact area of the femoral heads. The damage that was detected on some of these tapered neck specimens consistently occurred on the compression side. In Figures 2 and 3, a Scanning Electron Microscope (SEM) was used to show the medial contact area of two taper specimens. Figure 2 is a representative photograph of the medial aspect of a Co-Cr tested specimen showing some surface damage. Figure 3 is a representative photograph of the contact area of a Co-Cr untested specimen. The two comparative photographs in Figures 2 and 3 give a visual perspective of the degree of surface damage that was observed.

Visual inspection of the Ti-6Al-4V test specimens and corresponding femoral heads revealed no surface damage on the contact surface of the mating components. Figures 4 and 5 are a photographic comparison, taken from an SEM, which show the medial aspect of a Ti-6Al-4V tested specimen and a Ti-6Al-4V untested specimen.

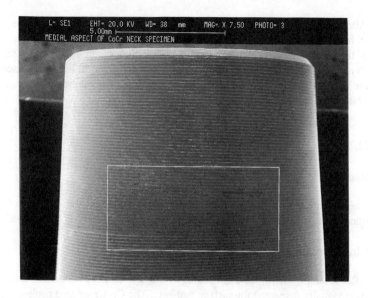

Fig. 2--SEM Photograph of the Medial Aspect of a Co-Cr Tested Specimen

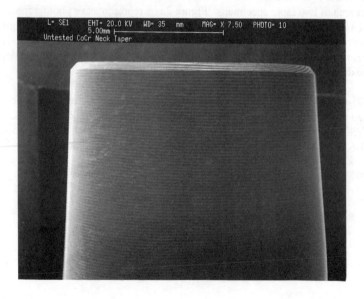

Fig. 3--SEM Photograph of the Medial Aspect of a Co-Cr Untested Specimen

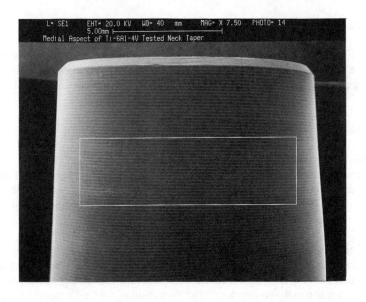

Fig. 4--SEM Photograph of the Medial Aspect of a Ti-6Al-4V Tested Specimen

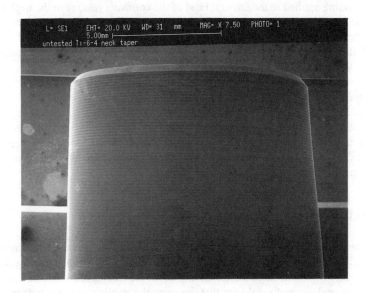

Fig. 5--SEM Photograph of the Medial Aspect of a Ti-6Al-4V Untested Specimen

Ion Release Analysis

The Ti ion release measurements for the test components were lower than the detectable limits (< 0.05 mg/L). The mean Co ion release measurements for similar and mixed metal components were 1.16±0.57 mg/L and 0.95±0.23 mg/L, respectively.

DISCUSSION

This testing methodology facilitates the assessment of design variables, manufacturing techniques, and other factors that can affect the performance of the femoral head/neck taper junction. The focus of this study is to characterize the fretting and wear debris generation for constructs of identical design consisting of Co-Cr and Ti-6Al-4V neck tapers in conjunction with Co-Cr femoral heads.

After all ten specimens had successfully completed ten million cycles, the femoral heads were disengaged and each construct was visually inspected. The inspection revealed that the Ti-6Al-4V tapered neck specimens and their mating femoral heads had no surface damage to the contact area. The inspection of the Co-Cr tapered neck specimens revealed that there was minor surface damage on some components. Most of the damage that was observed involved the deformation of the machined surface due to the relative micromotion between the femoral head and neck taper. It is believed that the off-axis loading applied to the femoral head of the construct relative to the neck taper axis causes the head to rock or pivot as the load is increased. The rocking or pivoting of the femoral head was probably less evident in the Ti-6Al-4V due to the flexion of the material allowed greater contact under this loading condition. No surface damage was visible in the mating femoral heads of the Co-Cr neck tapers.

The ion release data showed that similar metal constructs had a higher concentration of Co ions than the mixed metal constructs. The slightly higher concentration of Co ions can be attributed to the mild surface damage that was observed on the similar metal neck taper specimens as compared to mixed metal neck taper specimens. However, a T-test statistical analysis (P<0.05) found no significant difference in the measured ions for the two construct types.

SUMMARY AND CONCLUSION

In orthopaedics, the most popular modular connection is between the femoral head and nexk taper. Issues and implications regarding morse taper connections are still unclear today. With increased understanding about the mechanics of Morse taper connections, and test methodologies that can asses the stability of this interface accurately, a stable modular interface can be produced that will contribute to the longevity of total hip implants.

This study provides a method to evaluate the wear characteristics of the modular femoral head and the neck taper under fatigue. By using neck taper specimens, isolation of the head/neck interface is accomplished via a simple model of the morse taper connection. For this study, it was determined that the difference in the wear debris generated between the mixed metal and similar metal components of the same design was statistically insignificant.

REFERENCES

[1]   Gilbert, J.L., "Degradation in Modular Femoral Hip Prosthesis Tapers." NIH Consensus Development Conference on Total Hip Replacement, 1994, pp. 49-53.

[2]   Collier, J.P.; Surprenant, V.A.; Jenson, R.E.; and Mayor, M.D., "Corrosion at the Interface of Cobalt-Alloy Heads on Titanium-Alloy Stems." Clinical Orthopaedic Related Research, 271, 1991, pp. 305-312.

[3]   Bauer, T.W., Brown, S.A., Jiang, M., Panigutti, M.A., and Flemming, C.A.C., "Corrosion in Modular Hip Stems." Transactions of the 38th Annual ORS, Feb. 1992, p. 354.

[4]   McKellop, H.A., Sarmiento, A., Brien, W., and Park, S.H., "Interface Corrosion of a Modular Head Total Hip Prosthesis." Journal of Arthroplasty, 7 (3) 1992, pp. 291-294.

[5]   Dujovne, A.R., Bobyn, J.D., Krygier, J.J., Wilson, D.R., and Brooks, C.E., "Fretting at the Head/Neck Taper of Modular Hip Prosthesis." Transactions of the 4th World Biomaterials Congress, Berlin, Germany, April 1992, p. 264.

[6]   Lieberman, J.R., Rimnac, C.M., Garvin, K.L., Klien, R.W., and Salvati, E.A., "An Analysis of the Head-Neck Taper Interface in Retrieved Hip Prosthesis." Clinical Orthopaedic Related Research, 300, 1994, pp. 162-167.

[7]   International Standard ISO 7206-3 Part 3, Determination of the endurance properties of stemmed femoral components without the application of torsion. (1988-06-15).

[8]   Rohrle, H., Scholten, R., Sigolotto, C., Sollbauch, W., and Kellner, H., "Joint Forces in the Human Pelvis-Leg During Walking." Journal of Biomechanics, 17 (6), 1984, pp. 409-424.

[9]   Hardt, D.E., "Determining Muscle Forces in the Leg During Normal Human Walking-An Application and Evaluation of Optimization Methods." Journal of Biomechanical Engineering, 100 (2), 1978, pp. 72-78.

Andrew H. Schmidt,[1] Deb A. Loch,[2] Joan E. Bechtold,[3] and Richard F. Kyle[4]

ASSESSING MORSE TAPER FUNCTION : THE RELATIONSHIP BETWEEN IMPACTION FORCE, DISASSEMBLY FORCE, AND DESIGN VARIABLES

REFERENCE: Schmidt, A. H., Loch, D. A., Bechtold, J. E., and Kyle, R. F., "Assessing Morse Taper Function: The Relationship Between Impaction Force, Disassembly Force, and Design Variables," *Modularity of Orthopedic Implants, ASTM STP 1301,* Donald E. Marlowe, Jack E. Parr, and Michael B. Mayor, Eds., American Society for Testing and Materials, 1997.

ABSTRACT: Increasing experience with modular total hip implants has revealed problems with the Morse taper, including disassembly, corrosion, and wear debris. There are no standards for taper dimensions, manufacturing tolerances, or surface finish, and it is not known how these variables affect the function of the tapered connection. In this study, the relationship between the pull-off strength of a Morse taper and the force of impaction was determined for several commercial hip implants. The purpose of this study is to introduce this method of assessing Morse taper function, and to relate differences in taper performance to different design variables among the manufacturers. The results showed that taper distraction strength varies more than two-fold among the devices tested. Because of the many design differences noted among the different implants, the relative importance of each cannot be determined. Further work is warranted to refine these findings, and to identify the clinical significance of differences in taper distraction strength.

KEYWORDS: femoral component, modularity, Morse taper, total hip arthroplasty

[1]Faculty, Dept. of Orthopaedic Surgery, Hennepin County Medical Center, 701 Park Ave., Minneapolis, MN 55415.

[2]Orthopaedic Biomechanics Laboratory, Hennepin County Medical Center, 701 Park Ave. S., Minneapolis, MN 55415

[3]Orthopaedic Biomechanics Laboratory, Hennepin County Medical Center, 701 Park Ave. S., Minneapolis, MN 55415

[4]Chairman, Dept. of Orthopaedic Surgery, Hennepin County Medical Center, 701 Park Ave., Minneapolis, MN 55415.

Contemporary total hip arthroplasty is performed with modular devices that consist of a femoral stem and head joined by a tapered interlock (Morse taper) that is assembled intraoperatively. Clinical experience has shown that the Morse taper can function well for as long as ten-years. However, increasing follow-up has revealed many potential problems [1, 2], including component disassembly [3, 4] and corrosion [2, 5, 6, 7, 8, 9, 10, 11, 12, 13, 14, 15, 16)]. The tapered interlock has also been shown to generate significant quantities of wear debris [14, 17, 18, 19, 20], which contributes to osteolysis about total joint implants [19] and is the most significant problem affecting the longevity of these devices [21].

There is no industry standard or consensus regarding taper dimensions, manufacturing tolerances, or surface finish [22]. Therefore, Morse tapers of different total hip implants have variable geometry, different degrees of taper angle mismatch, and surfaces that are not uniform. The clinical significance of these differences is not known. The assessment of taper function can be made by either static testing (measuring the load to failure in distraction or torsion) or by fatigue testing. Clearly, static tests are easier to perform, and more information about the relative behavior of different tapers subjected to simple pull-off testing is needed. The purpose of the present study is to determine the degree of Morse taper design variability that exists among current prostheses, and to relate such differences to the mechanical strength of the taper as determined by distraction testing.

In this study, the relationship between the pull-off strength of a Morse taper and the force of impaction was determined for several commercial hip implants. The purpose of this report is to introduce this method of assessing Morse taper function, and to relate differences in taper performance to different design variables among the manufacturers.

EXPERIMENTAL METHOD

Taper Characterization.

Commercially available, modular total hip implants were obtained from four manufacturers. Stems were titanium alloy and the heads cobalt-chrome alloy with a 28 mm diameter and neutral neck length. Five pairs of each type were received and sent to an independent laboratory (National Calibration and Testing Labs, Minneapolis, MN) for measurement of taper geometry and surface roughness. Measurements of taper height and diameter were made with a touch-probe device capable of resolving distances of 1.3 micrometres (50 millionths of an inch). Taper angles were then calculated using standard formulae (Fig. 1). Five repeated meaurements of the same taper showed a standard error of 0.02 degrees.

Taper Assembly.

For each type of implant, four head/neck pairs were tested. Taper pairs were selected after review of their dimensions. One pair was chosen to have the maximum positive (neck larger than bore) taper angle mismatch, and a second pair chosen to have the greatest negative (neck smaller than bore) taper angle mismatch. A third pair was selected to have the minimum taper angle mismatch possible. The fourth pair was made at random. A fifth pair was left untested to serve as a control specimen for possible analysis of surface finish.

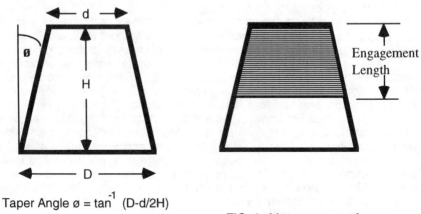

Taper Angle $\varnothing = \tan^{-1} (D\text{-}d/2H)$

FIG. 1--Calculation of Taper Angle

FIG. 2--Measurement of Engagement Length

The tapers were assembled in such a way as to provide a uniform impaction force that is similar to that used in clinical practice, using a drop tower. This methodology has been used in earlier studies [23]. Testing was performed in dry conditions at room temperature. For each taper pair, the relationship between impaction force and distraction force was measured as follows: The taper was positioned vertically in a rigid fixture beneath a drop tower manufactured from PVC pipe, with a standard femoral head impactor placed on the femoral head. A 1.4 kg cylindrical weight, held within the drop tower, was dropped from varying heights onto the impactor. The assembled implant was then mounted in a self-centering universal hinge fixture, and the head pulled axially off of the stem with a linear materials testing device (Enduratec Systems, Eden Prairie, MN). The distraction force applied was a ramp load of 450 kg/sec. Testing was performed by changing the height at which the weight was dropped by 2.54 cm (1 in.) intervals. For each implant, the testing was performed repeatedly (40 to 60 tests), with the drop height incremented in both ascending and in descending order. The pull-off strength was recorded at each interval, and the next test immediately performed.

Evaluation of the taper surfaces at the conclusion of testing showed clear scratching of all of the femoral components. For taper types A, C, and D, there was a distinct demarcation between the scratched area and the normal taper surface near the base. This distance of this line from the tip of the taper was felt to represent the engagement length of the taper and was measured with a hand-held digital caliper (Mitutoyo Model CD-6 BS, resolution 0.01 mm, error ± 0.02 mm, repeatability 0.01 mm) and recorded for each taper pair (Fig. 2). The ridges on the surface of taper B made the surface scratches very indistinct, and this measurement was not possible for taper type B.

Data pairs, consisting of the height at which the weight was dropped and the corresponding pull-off force, were plotted and analyzed by first-order linear regression. Regression coefficients were compared among the different pairs using one-way analysis of variance (ANOVA) and step-wise unpaired t-tests. Statistical significance is considered to represent $p \leq 0.05$. For the step-wise comparison of the 4 groups, the Bonferroni correction was utilized and statistical significance set at $p \leq 0.0083$.

RESULTS

Taper Geometry:

Design parameters differed among the four taper types. Mean values for the four pairs of each of the four types of tapers are shown in Table 1. Tapers from manufacturers A and D had smooth surfaces with a roughness of 0.41 and 0.30 micrometres, respectively. Companies B and C machine ridges into the surface of the femoral component, causing a marked increase in the roughness to greater than 1.73 micrometres. The finish of the taper surface within the femoral heads was smooth for all types with roughness varying between 0.20 and 0.51 micrometres (Table 1).

TABLE 1--Taper dimensions.

Taper	Stem angle (deg) (mean ± S.D.)	Stem range (deg.)	Stem rough-ness (μm)	Head angle (deg) (mean ± S.D.)	Head Range (deg.)	Head Rough-ness (μm)
A	3.00 ± 0.00	2.99-3.00	0.41	2.99 ± 0.01	2.99-3.00	0.41
B	2.82 ± 0.01	2.81-2.83	2.03	2.88 ± 0.00	2.87-2.88	0.20
C	2.83 ± 0.01	2.81-2.83	1.73	2.83 ± 0.03	2.79-2.88	0.51
D	1.50 ± 0.00	1.49-1.51	0.30	1.49 ± 0.01	1.47-1.51	0.41

Taper angles were consistent among prostheses of a given type but differed depending on the manufacturer (Table 1). With the exception of manufacturer B, the taper angles generally matched within the range of tolerances. Prosthesis B had a consistent taper angle mismatch with the angle of the femoral stem smaller (straighter) than the head, leading to contact within the depth of the taper and potential opening at the mouth of the taper.
The engagement length of the taper is also a function of taper dimension and was measured for each taper pair (Table 2). Examination of the engagement length shows that the distance was identical within the precision of measurement for all implants from manufacturers A and C. The engagement length for taper D was variable for the four specimens tested. Inspection of the surfaces also showed that the scratching was very uniform and homogeneous for taper types A and C, whereas the scratching of type D was patchy and inconsistent. This implies consistently large surface area contact among types A and C, and lesser, more variable amounts of contact for type D.

TABLE 2--Engagement length.

Taper	Engagement Length (mm)
A1	12.70
A2	12.70
A3	12.70
A4	12.70
B1	-
B2	-
B3	-
B4	-
C1	16.13
C2	16.13
C3	16.13
C4	16.13
D1	13.73
D2	12.85
D3	15.01
D4	15.42

Pull-off Force:

Evaluation of the raw data shows that pull-off force is an increasing function of the impaction force, and is well represented by a straight line (Figs. 3-6). Standard linear regression techniques were used to determine the regression coefficients for each prosthesis (Table 3). Comparison of all of the regression lines for a given type of prosthesis plotted on common axes showed that the lines tended to group together. The data for all taper pairs of a given prosthetic design were therefore pooled so that a single first order linear regression line was determined for each manufacturer (Figs. 3-6).

Statistical analysis of the regression coefficients was performed in order to attempt to support the observation that the prostheses differed among manufacturers. As shown in Table 3, the regression equation was used to estimate the pull-off force at a height of 35 cm. This value was chosen to represent the constant term since it is in the mid-range of the heights used and the regression lines do not actually intersect the ordinate axis. The derived constant and the slopes of the various lines were then compared using one-way ANOVA for 4 groups. The slopes were shown to differ significantly among the 4 types ($F=4.3$, $0.01 < p \leq 0.025$). The constant varied even more significantly ($F=19.7$, $p \leq 0.001$). Step-wise, unpaired t-tests showed significant differences between the constants of types A/B ($p \leq 0.005$) and A/D ($p \leq 0.005$). The other individual comparisons of constants were not significant: A/C = $0.1 < p \leq 0.25$, B/C = $0.05 < p \leq 0.1$, B/D = $0.01 < p \leq 0.025$, and C/D = $0.005 < p \leq 0.01$. Similar step-wise comparisons of the slopes did not reach statistical significance for any pair of regression lines.

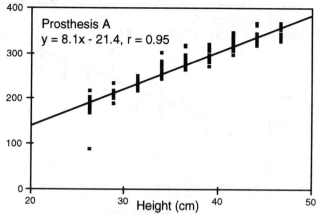

FIG. 3--Pooled data for taper type A.

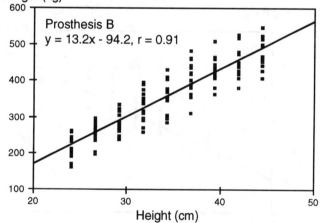

FIG. 4--Pooled data for taper type B.

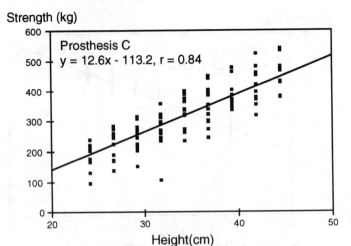

FIG. 5--Pooled data for taper type C.

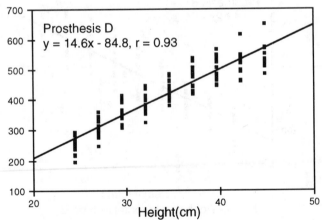

FIG. 6--Pooled data for taper type D.

TABLE 3--Linear Regression Coefficients

Prosthesis	Constant	Slope	Pull-off Force @ 35 cm	Coefficient of correlation
A1	1.5	7.5	264.0	.95
A2	-9.8	7.8	263.2	.98
A3	-32.8	8.2	254.2	.98
A4	-44.5	8.9	267.0	.94
B1	-109.7	14.4	394.3	.92
B2	-121.4	13.3	344.1	.97
B3	-79.4	12.7	365.1	.97
B4	-65.0	12.3	365.5	.86
C1	-84.2	11.7	325.3	.85
C2	-162.7	14.5	344.8	.88
C3	-92.6	11.6	313.4	.83
C4	-34.0	7.4	225.0	.96
D1	-98.8	15.7	450.7	.97
D2	-55.2	12.9	396.3	.97
D3	-114.2	14.9	407.3	.98
D4	-147.4	17.6	468.6	.95

In order to facilitate comparison the four regression lines (with associated 95% confidence limits) described above are plotted on a common set of axes in Fig. 7.

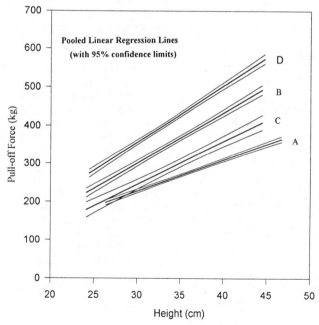

FIG. 7--Linear regression lines: impaction height versus pull-off force

DISCUSSION

Orthopaedic industry standards for the specification of Morse tapers are nonexistent, and typical medical taper tolerances are eight-fold lower than those used in the automotive and machine tool industries [24]. Retrieval studies have shown that certain prosthetic types are more prone to fretting and corrosion than others, suggesting that design factors may be significant [25, 26]. However, very few studies have specifically examined the relationship of taper dimension and function. It has been shown that taper angle mismatch causes increased fretting [6, 27]. Alexander and Noble [28] studied the torsional fatigue strength of a series of tapers and showed that the load to failure was also related to the amount of taper angle mismatch. Cook et al. [14] performed a similar fatigue study and found that tapers with a greater angle mismatch generated more particulate debris than more congruent tapers. Bobyn et al. [18] analyzed three different prosthetic designs and found that the Morse tapers in all three produced large quantities of particulate debris. However, the differences were not related specifically to taper design in the latter study.

Clinically, osteolysis is now considered to be the primary problem affecting the longevity of prosthetic joints [21]. Osteolysis appears to be the end result of a cascade of events that result from the accumulation of particulate matter of any type, including metallic debris, polyethylene particles, or fragmented bone cement [19]. Since wear debris provides the impetus for the clinical phenomenon of osteolysis, it becomes imperative to understand and minimize the potential sources of wear debris. Morse tapers have been shown to generate particulate debris. Design factors that may influence debris formation within Morse tapers are poorly understood and need more research.

This study highlights the different design philosophies apparent among four manufacturers (Table 1). Two stems (A,D) had smooth surfaces (Ra 0.30-0.41 micrometres) while two others (B,C) had ridged surfaces (Ra 1.73-2.03 micrometres). Absolute taper angles varied, as did the degree of taper angle mismatch. With respect to the pull-off strength, data were reproducible for a given implant. This reproducibility was not affected by repeated testing or whether the testing was done in an increasing or decreasing fashion. The data were also reproducible for the ridged devices (tapers B and C) which might be expected to deform during testing. Regression lines representing the relationship between taper impaction force and resistance to disassembly vary significantly between the different devices tested (Fig. 7). Because of the numerous variables present, the relative influence of a given design parameter on taper strength is not known. However, based on these data, it appears that a smaller taper angle improves the distraction strength (compare Taper D versus A,B,C). The addition of ridges alone does not seem to be sufficient to improve strength (compare Taper A versus Taper C). The effect of taper angle mismatch can be assessed in two ways. First, prostheses B and C (Table 1) differ primarily in the larger bore angle in type B. This type of taper mismatch leads to point contact at the tip of the stem and does seem to improve taper strength. Secondly, the effect of manufacturing tolerances dictates that even among prostheses of the same type, there will be varying degrees of taper mismatch (Table 2). However, there was not any consistent relationship between intra-manufacturer mismatch and taper strength, probably because other design tolerances were also randomly varying. The final parameter evaluated was the engagement length of the taper. Prostheses A and C had identical engagement lengths for all four pairs, whereas prosthesis D had highly variable engagement lengths. Comparison of the engagement length of the taper types and their relative strengths failed to show any direct correlation, showing that other design features are likely more important.

We have shown that commercial total hip implants from different manufacturers have distinct design differences that affect taper function. Taper distraction strength varies more than two-fold among these devices for comparable impaction forces. Further work is warranted to refine these findings, and to identify the clinical significance of differences in taper distraction strength. Standardized taper testing protocols and manufacturing should contribute to improved clinical results with these devices.

REFERENCES

[1]   Barrack R. L., Burke D. W., Cook S.D., et al., "Complications Related to Modularity of Total Hip Components," The Journal of Bone and Joint Surgery, **75B**: 688-92, 1993.

[2]   Collier, J. P., Mayor, M. B., Williams, I. R., Surprenant, V. A., Surprenant, H. P., and Currier, B. H., "The Tradeoffs Associated with Modular Hip Prostheses," Clinical Orthopaedics and Related Research, **311**: 91-101, 1995.

[3]   Pellicci, P. M., and Haas, S.B., "Disassembly of a Modular Femoral Component During Closed Reduction of the Dislocated Femoral Component: a Case Report," The Journal of Bone and Joint Surgery, **72A**: 619-620, 1990.

[4]   Woolson, S. T., and Pottorff, G. T., "Disassembly of a Modular Femoral Prosthesis After Dislocation of the Femoral Component: a Case Report," The Journal of Bone and Joint Surgery, **72A**: 624-625, 1990.

[5]   Bauer, T. W., Brown, S. A., Jiang, M., Panigutti, M. A., and Flemming, C.A.C., "Corrosion in Modular Hip Stems," Transactions 38th Annual Meeting, Orthopaedic Research Society, Feb. 17-20, 1992, p. 354.

[6]   Brown, S. A., Flemming, C. A. C., Kawalec, J. S., Vassaux, C. J., Payer, J. H., Kraay, M. J., and Merritt, K., "Fretting Accelerated Crevice Corrosion of Modular Hips," Transactions Implant Retrieval Symposium, Society for Biomaterials, Sept. 17-20, 1992, p. 59.

[7]   Buckley, C. A., Gilbert, J. L., Urban, R. M., Sumner, D. R., Jacobs, J. J., and Lautenschlager, E.P., "Mechanically Assisted Corrosion of Modular Hip Prosthesis Components in Mixed and Similar Metal Combinations," Transactions Implant Retrieval Symposium, Society for Biomaterials, Sept. 17-20, 1992, p. 58.

[8]   Collier, J. P., Surprenant, V. A., Jensen, R. E., and Mayor, M. B., "Corrosion at the Interface of Cobalt-alloy Heads on Titanium-alloy Stems," Clinical Orthopaedics and Related Research, 271: 305-312, 1991.

[9]   Collier, J. P., Surprenant, V. A., Mayor, M. B., and Jensen, R. E., "Corrosion and Fracture of All-cobalt-alloy Hip Prostheses," Transactions Implant Retrieval Symposium, Society for Biomaterials, Sept. 17-20, 1992, p. 62.

[10]   Collier, J. P., Surprenant, V. A., Jensen, R. E., Mayor, M. B., and Surprenant, H. P., "Corrosion Between the Components of Modular Femoral Hip Prostheses," The Journal of Bone and Joint Surgery, 74B: 511-5517, 1992.

[11]   Collier, J. P., Surprenant, V. A., Mayor, M. B., Jensen, R. E., and Surprenant, H.P., "Corrosion of Mixed-alloy Femoral Hip Components," Transactions Implant Retrieval Symposium, Society for Biomaterials, Sept. 17-20, 1992, p. 60.

[12]   Collier, J. P., Surprenant, V. A., Mayor, M. B., Jensen, R. E., and Surprenant, H. P., "Corrosion of the Head/neck Taper of Modular Femoral Hip Components," Orthopaedic Transactions, 16(1): 1992.

[13]   Collier, J. P., Mayor, M. B., Jensen, R. E., Surprenant, V. A., Surprenant, H. P., McNamara, J. L., and Belec, L., "Mechanisms of Failure of Modular Prostheses," Clinical Orthopaedics and Related Research, 285: 129-139, 1992.

[14]   Cook, S. D., Barrack, R. L., Baffes, G. C., et al., "Wear and Corrosion of Modular Interfaces in Total Hip Replacements," Clinical Orthopaedics and Related Research, 298: 80-88, 1994.

[15]   Mathiesen, E. B., Lindgren, J. U., Blomgren, G. G. A., and Reinholt, F. P., "Corrosion of Modular Hip Prostheses," The Journal of Bone and Joint Surgery, 73B: 569-575, 1993.

[16]   McKellop, H. A., Sarmiento, A., Brien, W., and Park, S. H., "Interface Corrosion of a Modular Head Total Hip Prosthesis," The Journal of Arthroplasty, 7: 291-294, 1992.

[17]   Baffes, G. C., Cook, S. D., Kester, M. A., Dong, N., and Serekian, P.,
        "Wear and Corrosion of Modular Interfaces in Total Hip Replacements,"
        Transactions 20th Annual Meeting of the Society for Biomaterials, April 5-
        9, 1994, p. 458.

[18]   Bobyn, J. D., Tanzer, M., Krygier, J.J., et al., "Concerns with Modularity in
        Total Hip Arthroplasty," Clinical Orthopaedics and Related Research, 298:
        27-36, 1994.

[19]   Urban, R. M., Jacobs, J. J., Gilbert, J. L., and Galante, J.O., "Corrosion
        Products of Modular Hip Prostheses: Microchemical Identification and
        Histopathological Significance," Transactions 39th Annual Meeting,
        Orthopaedic Research Society, Feb. 15-18, 1993, p. 81.

[20]   Urban R. M., Jacobs J. J., Gilbert J. L., and Galante J. O., "Migration of
        Corrosion Products From Modular Hip Prostheses: Particle Microanalysis
        and Histopathological Findings," The Journal of Bone and Joint Surgery,
        76A: 1345-59, 1994.

[21]   Harris W.H., "The Problem is Osteolysis," Clinical Orthopaedics and
        Related Research, 311: 46-53, 1995.

[22]   Skinner, H.B., "Current Biomaterials Problems in Implants," In AAOS
        Instructional Course Lectures, ed. Robert E. Eilert, Vol. XLI, Chapter 14,
        pp. 137-139, 1992.

[23]   Loch, D. A., Gleason, K. A., Kyle, R. F., and Bechtold, J.E., "Axial Pull-off
        Strength of Dry and Wet Taper Head Connections on a Modular Shoulder
        Prosthesis," Presented at Orthopaedic Research Society, Feb. 22, 1994.

[24]   Dujovne, A. R., Bobyn, J. D., Krygier, J. J., Young, D. L., and Brooks, C.
        E., "Surface Analysis of the Taper Junctions of Retrieved and In-Vitro
        Tested Modular Hip Prostheses," Transactions 19th Annual Meeting of the
        Society for Biomaterials, April 28-May 2, 1993, p. 276.

[25]   Justice, T. A., Lucas, L. C., and Lemons, J. E., "Investigations of 2-15
        Year Retrieved Ti-6Al-4V/Co-Cr-Mo Total Hip Prostheses," Transactions
        Implant Retrieval Symposium, Society for Biomaterials, Sept. 17-20, 1992,
        p. 57.

[26]   Sauer, W., Kovacs, P., Beals, N.,and Cuckler, J., "Corrosion at Head/taper
        Interfaces: A 3-5 Year Follow-up of Modular Head/Ti-6Al-4V Femoral Stem
        Prostheses," Transactions Implant Retrieval Symposium, Society for
        Biomaterials, Sept. 17-20, 1992, p. 56.

[27]   Flemming, C. A. C., Brown, S. A., and Payer, J.H., "The Use of Fretting
        Currents to Examine the Issue of Tolerances in Modular Hips,"
        Transactions 19th Annual Meeting of the Society for Biomaterials, April 28-
        May 2, 1993, p. 275.

[28]   Alexander, J. W., and Noble, P. C., "The effect of taper mismatch on the torsional properties of conical joints," _Transactions 39th Annual Meeting, Orthopaedic Research Society_, Feb. 15-18, 1993, p. 436.

Herbert G. Richter[1], Gerd Willmann[2], Martin Wimmer[1], and Frank G. Osthues[1]

INFLUENCE OF THE BALL/STEM-INTERFACE ON THE LOAD BEARING CAPABILITY OF MODULAR TOTAL HIP ENDOPROSTHESES

REFERENCE: Richter, H. G., Willmann, G., Wimmer, M., and Osthues, F. G., "Influence of the Ball/Stem-Interface on the Load Bearing Capability of Modular Total Hip Endoprostheses," *Modularity of Orthopedic Implants, ASTM STP 1301,* Donald E. Marlowe, Jack E. Parr, and Michael B. Mayor, Eds., American Society for Testing and Materials, 1997.

ABSTRACT: An extremely high level of mechanical reliability is required of total hip joint replacement systems. The reliability has to be proven in part by testing for resistance to static load using test tapers. There is evidence that the load bearing capability of the ball/stem-system is influenced by the surface structure of the taper. However, no systematic investigation is available in which this influence is studied in more detail. In the present study the surface structure of metal tapers is varied systematically in order to evaluate the influence of groove depth and pitch on the resistance to static load. Test tapers were produced from both a Titanium-alloy and a Cobalt-Chrome-alloy. The test results show that the burst strength increases with increasing "deformability" of the metal taper surface structure. A simple formula is put forward for estimating of the "deformability".

KEYWORDS: Ceramic hip joint head, resistance to static load, burst strength, metal taper surface structure, Titanium-alloy, Cobalt-Chrome-alloy.

INTRODUCTION

In a study carried out in 1993 the strength bearing capability of zirconia hip joint heads (28 mm diameter, taper 12/14, long neck) was measured with commercially available test tapers [1]. Additional characteristics of the hip joint heads were an angle of $5°43'30'' +5'$, $-0'$, and a straightness deviation of $<3\mu m$. The metal test tapers were made to one single specification for the angle ($5° 42' 30'' +0'$, $-5'$), the straightness deviation ($<3\mu m$), and the roundness deviation ($<8 \mu m$). The surface structure of these tapers was according to the taper manufacturers specifications.

These test tapers were produced by different manufacturers from different alloys, namely from Ti-alloy Ti6Al4V (ISO 5832-3), from Cobalt-Chrome-alloy (ISO 5832-4) and from an alloy according to ISO 5832-6.

[1]CERASIV GmbH, R&D, Plochingen, Germany
[2]CERASIV GmbH, Medical Products Division, Plochingen, Germany

The results regarding the resistance to static load are shown in Fig. 1: The load bearing capability ranges from 50 to 110 kN; the CoCr-tapers (manufacturer B, D and F) are at the lower end of the strength distribution, whereas the Ti-alloy tapers (manufacturer H, C and G) are at the upper end. The highest strength was found with the CoNiCrMo-taper (manufacturer E).

An attempt to take into account the surface structure in terms of R_{max} results in a dependence shown in Fig. 2: The data for the Ti-alloy tapers lie on a curve which is significantly different from the curve for the CoCr-alloy tapers. Similar results were obtained when using other roughness parameters.

The result was not completely satisfactory in that it was not possible to find a material independent correlation between the strength data and roughness parameters. That means that additional parameters have to be taken into account.

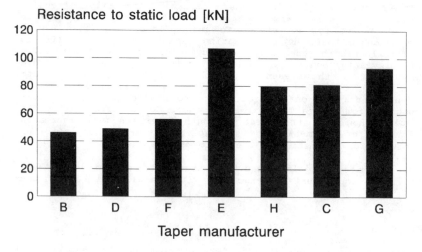

Resistance to static load [kN]

Taper manufacturer

FIG. 1-Resistance to static load (according to ISO 7206 part 5 [2]) of zirconia ceramic hip joint heads tested with various test tapers.

Therefore, an additional test program was set up in order to study the influence of systematically varied surface structures on the burst strength (resistance to static load) of alumina hip joint heads.

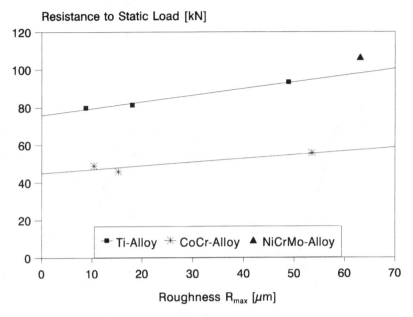

FIG. 2- Resistance to static load (according to ISO 7206 part 5) of zirconia ceramic hip joint heads as a function of R_{max} of the taper surface structure (after [1]).

EXPERIMENTAL METHOD

Out of the various potential surface structures a trapezoidal profile was chosen (Fig. 3). Threads with this profile were produced by standard machining processes utilizing a specially shaped tool. The depths of the grooves were chosen to be 15 µm, 45 µm and 60 µm, resp. The bottom width, b, was held constant at a width of 60 µm. The pitch (distance between grooves, p) was varied between 80 µm and 220 µm. Accordingly the plateau width, w, varied between 135 µm and 15 µm.

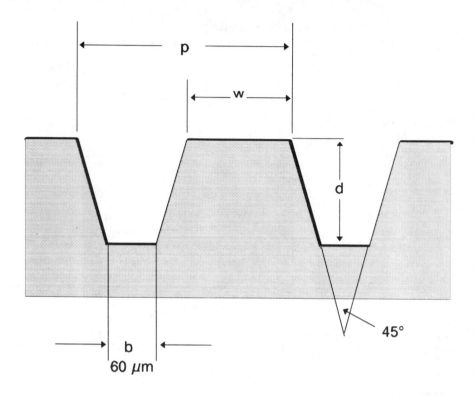

d = 15 μm, 45 μm, 60 μm
w= 80 μm ... 220 μm

FIG. 3-Schematic of the thread profile in experimental test tapers.

The burst strength of the taper/hip-joint-head-system was measured according to ISO 7206 part 5 using standard alumina hip joint heads with 28 mm diameter, 12/14 taper and long neck. Heads and tapers were produced to the geometry specifications described in the Introduction. For each set of material, groove depth and groove distance at least 10 strength experiments were run.

RESULTS

Fig. 4 gives the burst strengths in dependence on the pitch, p, as measured before the test. Each data point represents the average calculated from at least 10 burst strength experiments. In general, the standard deviation is around 8 % of the average, and the average values differ significantly from each other.

There is a wide range in burst strengths from around 40 kN for CoCr-alloy tapers up to above 90 kN for Ti-alloy tapers. These values lie in the range which is well documented for alumina hip joint balls of the type used in the present study [3], [4], [5].

There is a significant increase in strength with decreasing pitch. additional parameter is the depth of the grooves: the deeper the grooves the higher the load bearing capability of the taper/ball-system.

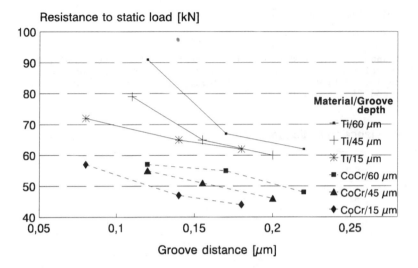

FIG. 4-Resistance to static load of alumina hip joint heads in dependence on the groove distance (pitch), p, and depth, d, on Ti-alloy and CoCr-alloy test tapers.

In the present study one sample of ball heads was used. The only parameters varied were the taper material (Ti-alloy and CoCr-alloy) and the surface structure of the taper. The working hypothesis is put forward, that in the present study the deformability of the surface profile is the controlling factor for the load bearing capability of the ball/stem-system. In contrast to the findings reported in [1] the dependence of the resistance to static load on the deformability can not be described satisfactorily by the quotient of hardness and roughness R_a (H/R_a), because the effect of the groove distance which is quite obvious in Fig. 4 is not considered in this relation.

It is suggested that an additional parameter has to be taken into account which describes the groove profile in more detail. Roughness parameters such as R_a or R_{max} are not appropriate parameters in this context because they would not provide an explicit characterization of the groove profile and, especially, of the pitch.

In order to describe the findings the real geometry of the profile has to be taken into account. So the data for d and p are not derived from diamond stylus profilometry but from cross-sections.

In a very simplistic way the deformability can be defined in terms of groove depth, d, width of the plateau between two grooves (measured before loading), w, and hardness, HV, in the following form

$$\text{Deformability} = \frac{d}{w \cdot HV} \tag{1}$$

where d = groove depth
       w = plateau width
       HV = Vickers hardness

Fig. 5 shows the dependence of the resistance to static load (burst strength) in relation to the "deformability" as defined by equation (1). The data are represented quite satisfactorily by a straight line with a correlation coefficient of 0.9.

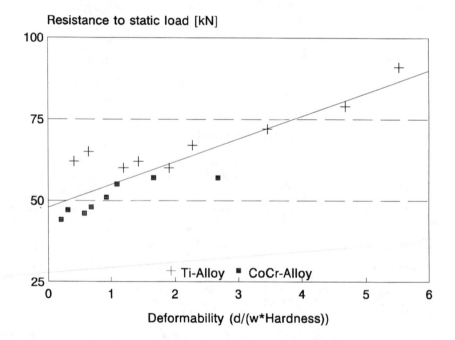

FIG. 5-Resistance to static load as a function of the deformability of the taper surface structure.

The conclusion has to be drawn that the load bearing capability of the taper/ball system is not completely described by the outer geometry and by a roughness parameter but that the real groove profile together with the material hardness must be taken into account.

REFERENCES

[1] Bachnik, M., Hasenpusch, M., et al, „The Effect of Hardness and Surface Quality of Metal Tapers on the Fracture Load of Ceramic Ball Heads in Hip Endoprostheses,‟ Biomedizinische Technik Vol. 39, No. 12, 1994, pp 302-306.

[2] ISO 7206 part 5: Implants for surgery. Partial and total hip joint prostheses. Part 5: Determination of resistance to static load of head and neck region of stemmed femoral components, 1992.

[3] Dörre, E., et al, „Fracture Load of Ceramic Ball Heads of Hip Joint Prostheses,‟ Biomediz. Technik Vol. 36, No. 12, 1991,m pp. 305-307.

[4] Willmann, G., „Das Prinzip der Konus-Steckverbindung für keramische Kugelköpfe bei Hüftendoprothesen,‟ Mat.-wiss. und Werkstofftechnik Vol. 24, 1993, pp 315-319.

[5] Heimke, G., The Safety of Ceramic Balls on Metal Stems in Hip Arthroplasty,‟ Advanced Materials Vol. 6, No. 2, 1994, pp. 165-170.

State of the Art in Properties Testing II

Michael B. Cooper,[1] Mary E. Anthony,[2] Abraham B Salehi,[3] ánd Jeff A. Holbrook[4]

FATIGUE INTEGRITY TEST OF A MODULAR TIBIAL STEM EXTENSION

REFERENCE: Cooper, M. B., Anthony, M. E., Salehi, A. B., and Holbrook, J. A., **"Fatigue Integrity Test of a Modular Tibial Stem Extension,"** *Modularity of Orthopedic Implants, ASTM STP 1301,* Donald E. Marlowe, Jack E. Parr, and Michael B. Mayor, Eds., American Society for Testing and Materials, 1997.

ABSTRACT: With the frequent use of modular knee systems today, component integrity at the modular interface is often questioned. Many knee systems use modular stem extensions that attach to the tibial or femoral component. The use of these modular stems raise issues about the fatigue integrity of the construct, fretting of the modular connection, and modular attachment strength. These must be addressed through testing in order to validate the safety and efficacy of a product. Three test methods that can be used to investigate the fatigue integrity of the modular tibial tray and stem interface will be discussed. The three test methods discussed are the Cantilever Test, the Unsupported Stem Test, and the Partial Bone Support Test. Each of these test methods is compared and contrasted on their ability to mimic clinical conditions, ease of use, and ease of analysis. The test methods attempt to address several issues relevant to modular tibial stem extensions. The presentation of the test methods is meant to provide information on current stem extension testing in order to fuel the emergence of a standardized testing protocol.

KEYWORDS: tibia, stems, modularity, test methods, fatigue

[1] Research Engineer II, device testing
[2] Research Engineer II, device testing
[3] Research Specialist, analysis
[4] Senior Research Technician, device testing, Technical Services, Smith & Nephew Richards Inc., 1450 Brooks Road, Memphis TN 38116.

INTRODUCTION

Orthopedic implants for use in total knee replacement (TKR) surgery have become increasingly more versatile in treating deformities and accommodating new demands for surgical intervention. This has been done through the use of modular components and accessories. Modular total knee systems can accommodate a variety of indications with one knee system without forcing the surgeon to foresee specific problems in advance. These systems allow for the use of a variety of different types of tibial articulating surfaces to be attached to one tibial tray. Also, the same tibial tray can use tibial wedges to provide support in areas exhibiting bone defects and can facilitate a number of different diameters, lengths, and shaped long stem extensions to provide additional stability for the tibial tray. Similar accessories also exist for the femoral component. One femoral component can accommodate long stem extension and femoral wedges. This degree of modularity provides the surgeon with a variety of choices to fill a surgical need, yet also brings about heightened concern for the safety issues involved with the use of such a system.

One of the greatest areas of concern from both a surgical and structural aspect is tibial components. Clinically, tibial trays have been shown to fail in a cantilever type loading configuration [1-5]. This type of loading may occur when either the medial or lateral side of the tibial tray loses bone support. This loss of support allows for the majority of the load on the unsupported side of the tray to be compensated by the tibial tray, with very little load distributed to the bone. Cantilever type failures occur in both modular and monolithic type components. With a modular tibial tray, there is not only a concern about cantilever type failures of the tray, but also concerns that reflect use of the tray with any of its accessories. One such area of concern is the use of the tibial tray with a long stem extension.

The stem extension on tibial trays is used for added stability. A stem may be used in cases where there is a lack of good bone stock in the patient's tibia, or there may be some type of bone deformity that does not allow for adequate stability of the tray without the stem attachment [6,7]. In the case of tibial trays used with stem extensions, there is not only a concern for the structural integrity of the tibial tray itself (i.e. cantilever loading) but there is also a concern of the structural integrity of the stem extension (i.e. breakage of the stem extension), structural integrity of the total construct, and the integrity of the connection of the stem to the tray (i.e., breakage at the connection point of the stem and tray, disengagement of the stem and tray connection, and fretting at the stem and tray connection). With these added concerns, the question as to how to evaluate the safety and efficacy of this construct becomes an issue. This paper will discuss three different test methods by which it may be possible to evaluate the integrity of the tibial tray/tibial stem construct.

TEST METHODS

Tibial stem extensions are connected to the tibial tray in several ways. Three of the most common methods to connect a stem extension to a tibial tray are i) a Morse taper, ii) a screw connection, or iii) a Morse taper with a through-bolt. The connection point is an area of major concern for the structural integrity of the construct. In order to evaluate the strength of the tibial tray/stem construct, a test method must be developed that will apply an anatomical load similar to that applied in vivo. The test method should address concerns about the modularity of the implant and should address failures that are representative of failures seen clinically. The test method should also have the capability to compare different construct designs. Three test methods that attempt to accomplish this are the Cantilever Test, the Unsupported Stem Test, and the Partial Bone Support Test. These test methods will be compared and contrasted. These methods are proposed so that the orthopedic community will develop a standardized test method to help determine the safety of tibial tray/tibial stem constructs.

Cantilever Test--The Cantilever Test is a simple test to set-up but the analysis involved is not trivial. The purpose of the cantilever test is to apply load to a stem extension that has been attached to the tibial tray and fixed in a cantilever beam type configuration. This test applies a bending moment to the tibial tray/stem connection point in an attempt to disassemble the connection or fracture the connection point. Figure 1 shows an example of a test set-up configuration. The tibial stem has been attached to the tibial tray, by following the proper surgical procedure outlined by the manufacturer's surgical technique manual. The tray and stem are then positioned so that the tray is resting on its side. The superior part of the tray is rigidly fixed with the remaining distal part of the construct unsupported in a cantilever beam type configuration. A compressive, sinusoidal fatigue load is applied to the distal part of the stem extension. By applying the load in this manner, the stem undergoes a certain amount of bending and the tibial tray/stem connection point undergoes severe bending loads.

While this test evaluates the integrity of the modular connection, there is a question as to how well the test mimics in vivo conditions and at what load the construct should survive. The conditions imposed upon the tibial/stem construct under a cantilever condition are indicative of the clinical situation where the tibia may have been over-reamed for the tibial stem such that there is not a tight fit between the implant and the canal of the tibia. This loose fit allows the tibial stem to move inside the bone canal and thus become lodged against one of the bone canal walls. Under these circumstances, the stem is subjected to a side bending load. The loss of bone support under the tray and the lodging of the stem extension against the bone canal allow the tray to transmit a bending force to the construct similar to that seen in the cantilever test. However, it is hard to determine what load is applied to the construct under this clinical condition; therefore, determining a fatigue load at which to run the test is difficult.

One method of determining this load is to strain gauge the construct in a cadaver or simulated bone and load the construct with a femoral component as would happen in vivo. This strain level can then be matched to a load that will create the same strain level in the Cantilever Test position. If the strain gauge method is used it is still necessary to know where the region of high strain is located so that a gauge can be placed in that location. This region is not always apparent. Therefore, finite element analysis (FEA) is often used to determine high strain areas.

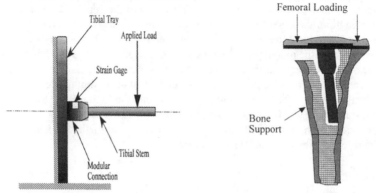

Figure 1.--Test Set-up Configuration (left) and Simulated Clinical Condition (right)

As can be seen, while the test set-up configuration for the Cantilever Test is simple, it does require a bit of effort to determine the appropriate load level suitable for testing the construct. Strain gauging, and FEA may be a part of this analysis routine. In addition to the difficulty in determining the proper test loads, this test also does not adequately test the entire construct as it would be used clinically. The issue of tibial tray fatigue is not addressed and would therefore still need to be assessed. In addition, it is unrealistic to think that the tibial stem does not undergo some type of axial loading in addition to the bending loads. Therefore, if the tibial stem was detached from the construct and the connection points examined visually for fretting after fatigue loading, the amount of fretting scars seen may not be indicative of the type of scars that would be seen under clinical loading conditions.

Unsupported Stem Test--In an attempt to test the tibial tray/tibial stem construct in a manner that more closely mimics in vivo conditions, the Unsupported Stem Test is proposed. One of the clinical conditions that may occur is the loss of bone support from the tibial tray. This has been seen in reported failures of tibial trays under cantilever loading conditions. The Unsupported Stem Test mimics complete bone loss from the tray and stem while loading the tibial construct eccentrically to also mimic a cantilevered loading condition on the tray. This test method will enable evaluation of the tibial tray, the tibial stem, and the tray/stem connection, all of which will undergo extreme bending loads.

For the test, the tibial stem extension should be attached to the tibial tray according to surgical procedure. The tibial construct should then be rigidly fixed such that only the distal-most point on the tibial stem extension is held rigid. The tray is then eccentrically loaded a certain distance from the anteroposterior and mediolateral centerline. A compressive, sinusoidal fatigue load should be applied to the construct, producing a load versus cycles to failure curve to determine fatigue integrity. A minimum of five constructs should be tested. Figure 2 shows the test set-up for this test method.

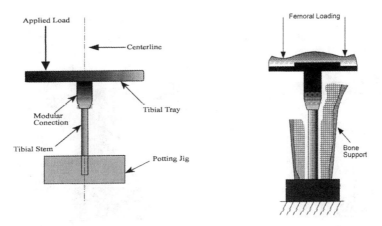

Figure 2.--Test Set-up Configuration (left) and Simulated Clinical Condition (right)

The advantage to this test method is that the tibial construct is loaded similarly to a worst case in vivo condition where an axial and bending load is applied to the construct. The loading is such that the construct may fail in either the tibial tray, tibial stem, or tibial tray/stem connection. By fixing the construct in the distal-most position, an extreme loss of bone support is modeled which allows extreme deformation of the stem during testing. This method also allows for the examination of the tray/stem connection for signs of fretting scars that may be more applicable to in vivo conditions. One of the biggest disadvantages of this test is that due to the extreme elastic deformation of the stem, the loading point often slips from its intended area, thus requiring constant adjustment of the set-up during the running of the test. Additionally, complete loss of bone support may represent overly harsh evaluation of the product in that a large amount of bone loss would probably lead to pain and require revision surgery long before the implant would fail.

Partial Bone Support--This test method is very similar to the test method for the Unsupported Stem Test except that this test is designed to represent a more realistic in vivo condition. This test mimics only a small amount of bone loss underneath the tibial tray, therefore supporting more of the stem extension and forcing more of the load to be distributed throughout the tray/stem connection and the tibial tray. This test still represents the cantilever loading conditions that have resulted in failures of tibial trays.

The Partial Bone Support Test requires that the stem extension be attached to the tibial tray by surgical procedure and be rigidly fixed some distance below the tray/stem connection juncture (i.e. 25 mm). This effectively mimics only a small amount of bone loss. The tray is eccentrically loaded some distance from the anteroposterior and mediolateral centerline. A compressive, sinusoidal fatigue load should be applied to the construct and a load versus cycle to failure curve should be developed to determine the fatigue integrity of the construct. Figure 3 shows the test set-up configuration.

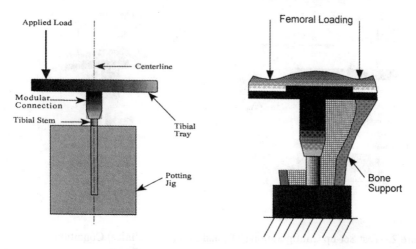

Figure 3.--Test Set-up Configuration (left) and Simulated Clinical Condition (right)

This test method more closely represents a severe in vivo condition in which the implant still must function. By limiting the amount of deflection that the stem was subjected to as with the unsupported stem test, the majority of the load can be distributed to the tray/stem connection and the tray. Thus, this test is harsher on the tray and the tray/stem juncture which are two of the major areas of concern. By loading the tray eccentrically, away from the tibial tray's centerline, the tibial tray is still subjected to cantilever loading conditions and the types of fractures seen in this type of configuration are consistent with the fractures reported clinically [1-5]. The stem extension can also be removed from the tibial tray after fatigue testing and the tray/stem connection can be inspected for fretting scars. These scars should be more representative of the type of fretting scars that would be seen under extreme in vivo conditions.

Other Stem Extension Concerns--Tibial stem extensions come in a variety of diameters and lengths, some are solid and some are slotted. While the difference in diameter sizes is meant to provide a press-fit fill of the bone canal, the difference in lengths and solid and slotted stems is meant not only to provide additional support for the tray in the presence of possible bone defects, but are to address the concerns of "end of stem" (tip) pain. This is hypothesized to be caused by a rigid diaphyseal stem extension making point contact with the lateral cortex of the tibia. Slotted stems are often used as an attempt to minimize this problem by decreasing the stiffness of the stem at the point of lateral contact with the tibial cortex.

Slotted stems may provide additional concerns as to the structural integrity of the stems. Slotted stems are made with slots of various lengths. The longer the slotted region, the more flexible the stem and thus the weaker the stem. Currently there is no guideline as to the maximum length of the slotted region. The slotted area of the stem must be sufficiently strong to resist the side loading it will experience at the point of contact with the tibial wall. While the load that the slots must withstand is presently unknown, the use of photoelastic analysis can provide some insight as to the amount of stress produced at the slotted stem region of the tibia. This stress level can then be used to make an educated guess as to the type of load at which the slotted stem should be tested. Testing of a special case stem extension such as this was not discussed in the test methods above. One test method that lends itself easily to determining the structural integrity of the slot is the Cantilever Test method. By using photoelasticity and strain gauging, the fatigue load can be determined. Alternatively, the Unsupported Stem Test can be used by rigidly fixing the stem extension with half of the slotted region exposed. This method applies a bending moment at the slotted region of the stem. It is the special cases such as the slotted stems for which an astute investigator must determine the proper loading criteria. The test methods outlined above were not meant to cover every special case stem and may need to be modified depending on the investigator's needs.

Additional Analysis Techniques--Some mention has already been made as to the use of additional analysis tools to support testing methodologies. In some instances it is difficult to know at what load to start a fatigue test so as to limit the amount of time and test specimens necessary to develop a load versus cycle to failure curve. Also, the structural problem areas in a test specimen are not readily apparent, nor in what test configuration the loading will be accurately applied to the test specimen. In instances such as these, it is often necessary to use additional analysis tools. One of the most cost effective analysis tools is finite element analysis (FEA). This method allows an engineer to computationally model the loading configuration of a test specimen and analyze the test specimen for problem areas, or predict fatigue endurance limits. FEA can show areas of high stress that predict where the component will fail under a loading configuration. This type of analysis is often helpful in determining a starting load at which to develop a load versus cycle to failure curve.

Another useful tool in representing a full field stress picture of a test specimen under a particular load condition is photoelastic analysis. This method allows the engineer to obtain a three-dimensional full field view of the stress field of a test specimen. This is often helpful in determining what type of loading configuration will distribute the loads in the area of concern.

One of the more frequently used tools is strain gauging. This analysis allows strain gauges to be applied directly to test specimens and allows evaluation of the strains in a component. This facilitates comparison of load-strain curves from the test conditions to in vivo conditions. A fatigue load can be determined which is considered reasonable for the survival of the construct. The problem with this analysis is that the engineer must know the area of concern in the implant to apply the gauge in the right area and in the right direction to obtain the maximum strain levels. In many instances it is still necessary to use FEA or photoelasticity to determine the area in which a strain gauge should be applied.

While some of the additional analyses may be slightly excessive, the investigator should not lose sight of the valuable information that can be obtained from these tools. Not only can a great deal be learned about a test method or the design of a component, but additional analysis methods can greatly improve the ability of a test to replicate conditions under which the test specimen should be tested. The investigator should always be cautious, however, in the use of these powerful analysis tools so as not to be led astray by the mountains of data that can be obtained.

CONCLUSIONS

All of these test methods were developed to address the potential concerns when using a modular stem extension and tibial tray. The Cantilever Test, while being simple to set-up, provides a challenge in determining proper loading requirements and provides an even greater challenge in determining exactly what the loading actually means in terms of conditions to which the implant will be subjected in vivo. The Unsupported Stem Test subjects the implant to more realistic in vivo conditions than what may have been achieved with the cantilever test. However, the deflections which the implant undergoes are unrealistic and an implant under such extreme bone loss conditions would more than likely undergo revision surgery. However, this test method does address the concerns of the integrity of the tibial tray under cantilever loading conditions while still addressing the concerns of the fatigue integrity of the tibial tray/stem juncture and the integrity of the construct as a whole. In addition, the tray/stem connection can be examined for fretting scars that would be similar to those inspected in vivo. The Partial Bone Support Test was meant to go one step further in the quest to more closely represent in vivo conditions. This test mimics only a small amount of bone loss to which the construct may be subjected and still addresses the concern of the fatigue integrity of the tibial tray, tray/stem connection, and overall integrity of the tray/stem construct. This test also distributes more loading to the tray/stem juncture and the tray thereby applying the load in the areas of major concern in a modular construct.

When using any of these test methods it may be necessary to use additional analysis techniques to properly evaluate the integrity of an orthopedic implant. Three of the most common analysis techniques are finite element analysis, photoelastic analysis, and strain gauging analysis. Any of these analyses can provide valuable information as to areas of an implant that are highly stressed or can be used to help ensure that a test method is actually applying the load to the test specimen in the manner in which the investigator designed. While the additional analysis is valuable, it can also lead the unwary investigator to erroneous decisions. Care should always be taken to properly analyze and understand the data before jumping to conclusions.

While these test methods were not meant to be all-inclusive, they were meant to provide information on current stem extension testing in order to help fuel the emergence of a standardized testing protocol. For each of these methods, there are probably another dozen variations that other investigators in the orthopedic industry are using. The emergence of a standardized testing protocol will enable the orthopedic industry to evaluate and compare designs in a consistent manner. One of the most important aspects in determining a proper protocol for this test is to try to closely imitate the in vivo loading condition in a fair and unbiased manner.

REFERENCES

[1]   Gradisar, I. A., Hoffman, B. S., and Askew, M. S., "Fracture of a Fenestrated Metal Backing of a Total Knee Component," Journal of Arthroplasty, Vol. 4, No. 1, March 1989, pp. 27-30.

[2]   Koeneman, J. B., Johnson, R. M., Weinstein, A. M., and Dupont, J. A., "Failure of Metal Tibial Trays," 12th Annual Meeting of the Society for Biomaterials, 1986, p. 146.

[3]   Mendes, D. G., Brando, D., Galor, R. L., and Roffman, M., "Breakage of the Metal Tray in Tibial Knee Replacements," Orthopedics, Vol. 7, No. 5, May 1984, pp. 860-862.

[4]   Morrey, B. F., and Chao, E. Y. S., "Fracture of the Porous-Coated Metal Tray of a Biologically Fixed Knee Prosthesis," Clinical Orthopedics and Related Research, No. 228, March 1988, pp. 182-189.

[5]   Scott, R. D., Ewald, F. C., and Walker, P. S., "Fracture of the Metallic Tibial Tray Following Total Knee Replacement: Report of Two Cases," Journal of Bone and Joint Surgery, Vol. 66A, June 1984, p. 780.

[6]   Mow, C. S., and Wiedel, J. D., "Noncemented Revision Total Knee Arthroplasty," Clinical Orthopedics and Related Research, No. 309, December 1994, pp. 110-115.

[7]   Murray, P. B., Rand, J. A., and Hanssen, A. D., "Cemented Long-Stem Revision Total Knee Arthroplasty," Clinical Orthopedics and Related Research, No. 309, December 1994, pp. 116-123.

Sushil K. Bhambri[1] and Leslie N. Gilbertson[1]

Fretting Corrosion Fatigue Study of Modular Joints in Total Hip Replacements by Accelerated *In Vitro* Testing

REFERENCE: Bhambri, S. K. and Gilbertson, L. N., "Fretting Corrosion Fatigue Study of Modular Joints in Total Hip Replacements by Accelerated *In Vitro* Testing," *Modularity of Orthopedic Implants, ASTM STP 1301,* Donald E. Marlowe, Jack E. Parr, and Michael B. Mayor, Eds., American Society for Testing and Materials, 1997.

ABSTRACT: The performance of modular head/taper joints in total hip replacements now in use for nearly two decades can be easily termed as a clinical success. However, associated with concerns of metal particulates found in retrieved tissues, a critical review of modularity in hip joints has recently emerged. Evaluation of retrieved modular joints has shown some surface morphological changes and debris generated at the mating surfaces which has not been demonstrated equally by any *in vitro* laboratory testing.

In this investigation, an experimental setup was developed to conduct fretting corrosion tests of modular head/taper assemblies in an aggressive environment to accelerate the *in vivo* phenomena. The fretting corrosion tests were conducted in a low pH Ringer's solution at 50°C. A maximum cyclic load of 5.34 kN was applied at 5 Hz on simulated modular head/ taper assemblies mounted in a 15° valgus anatomic orientation. Ti-6Al-4V and Co-Cr-Mo alloy tapers and Co-Cr-Mo alloy (cast or wrought) and zirconia ceramic femoral heads in various combinations were evaluated. The morphology evaluation of taper and head bore surfaces after 10 million cycles revealed features such as etching of structure, preferential leaching and fretting in congruence to those reported for retrieved modular hip joints. Nitrogen diffusion surface hardening of Ti-6Al-4V alloy tapers resulted in an increase in resistance to fretting corrosion-induced changes, and a reduction in generated debris. A zirconia ceramic femoral head tested on either a Ti-6Al-4V or a Co-Cr-Mo alloy taper showed an enhanced resistance to both mechanical and chemical phenomena.

KEYWORDS: fretting, corrosion, surface morphology, Ringer's solution, debris

INTRODUCTION

The modular femoral head/Morse taper joints in total hip replacements have gained a major share in surgical procedures in recent years. These modular joints offer a great flexibility in surgery in terms of component interchangeability and a reduced hospital inventory. The modular joints also allow selection of appropriate materials for the articulating surface (femoral head) and the load bearing component (hip stem) of the prosthesis. The strength requirement of the hip stem and wear resistance required for femoral head in total hip arthroplasty may necessitate dissimilar metal, metal/ceramic or similar metal components in the joint. These advantages of modular joints are not without concerns of their being a source of particulate debris *in vivo* [1] and fretting/crevice corrosion at the interfaces [2-7]. These concerns stem from the micromotion of modular components under physiological loading in aggressive body fluids. The absence, presence or severity of fretting and corrosion on taper and head-bore contact surfaces has been a subject of studies directed at understanding the effect of various factors such as geometry, chemistry, microstructure and surface properties of the contact surfaces of the modular joints.

---

[1]Senior research engineer and group manager, Engineering Test Laboratories, Zimmer, Inc. A wholly owned subsidiary of Bristol-Myers Squibb Company, P.O. Box 708, Warsaw, IN 46581-0708.

The similar or mixed metal modular head taper joints retrieved after several years of implantation have exhibited debris accumulated at the head/taper joints [4,5]. In addition, fretting/corrosion induced surface changes on both taper and bore contact surfaces were noticed on these retrievals. Gilbert et al. [6] observed etching of structure on the contact surface of Co-Cr-Mo femoral heads. Preferential leaching of a phase or element in the microstructure was also reported. The nature of these particles and their influence on the joint integrity *in vivo* have received greater attention recently, although no device explantation has been attributed to wear or corrosion of the modular head/taper joint. A few test methods developed have attempted to understand the mechanisms responsible in corrosion induced phenomena at the interfaces through electrochemical studies [6,8] or *in vitro* testing [9] but neither the debris generated nor the surface topographical changes in these studies replicated the retrieved devices.

In this study, fretting/corrosion phenomena during cyclic loading were accelerated to produce the *in vivo* effects by testing in low pH Ringer's solution at an elevated temperature, using a custom designed experimental setup. The test method was utilized to study the effect of nitrogen diffusion surface hardening of Ti-6Al-4V titanium alloy tapers on fretting corrosion behavior in couple with cast and wrought Co-Cr-Mo alloy and zirconia ceramic femoral heads.

MATERIALS AND METHODS

Morse taper cones simulating a hip stem taper were machined from wrought Ti-6Al-4V titanium alloy and Co-Cr-Mo alloy. These tapers had an average surface roughness Ra of 50 μm. Some of the Ti-6Al-4V alloy tapers were hardened by a low temperature nitrogen diffusion hardening process, *Ti-Nidium*™ Surface Hardening Process.* All taper cones were passivated following ASTM Standard F 86 prior to testing. The femoral heads were either cast or wrought Co-Cr-Mo alloy or zirconia ceramic and were obtained as commercial parts.

A customized experimental setup was designed and fabricated for conducting fretting corrosion tests on modular head taper assemblies mounted in 15° valgus stem orientation in an aggressive Ringer's solution (Fig. 1). A test setup constructed by Bhambri and Gilbertson [9] for fretting corrosion studies of modular head/taper joints was further developed for conducting tests in acidic Ringer's solution maintained at an elevated temperature of 50°C. The environmental chamber was made of Ti-6Al-4V titanium alloy lined with polyethylene on the inside and fitted with heating elements on the outside. The environmental chamber was connected to a distilled water reservoir for continuous replenishment of Ringer's solution evaporated during testing. Acidic Ringer's solution was prepared to a pH of 3.5 and filled in the chamber to a level covering the head/neck joint but below the poly acetal block used for applying load to the femoral head. The pH of the solution was monitored every day during the length of the test by using pH paper.

The femoral heads were assembled on the taper cones by applying 2.0 kN load axially on the heads. In case of metal heads, 32 mm long neck cobalt-chromium-molybdenum (Co-Cr-Mo) alloy heads were used for testing on both Ti-6Al-4V and Co-Cr-Mo alloy tapers. Zirconia ceramic femoral heads tested were 28 mm in diameter with a medium neck length. The fatigue load was applied on the femoral head by using a poly acetal block. A maximum cyclic load of 5.34 kN, six times the body weight of a 0.89 kN person, was applied to the femoral heads at a stress ratio of 0.1 and a frequency of 5 Hz.

Various head taper combinations used in this study are shown in Table 1. Five samples of each of the metal head/metal taper combinations were tested. In cases of ceramic head/metal taper modular joints, the zirconia ceramic femoral heads on three each of the Ti-6Al-4V alloy and Co-Cr-Mo alloy tapers were tested. The primary interest in this investigation was to determine the difference in fretting corrosion behavior of cast and wrought Co-Cr-Mo alloy heads and to determine the effect of nitrogen surface hardening on the fretting corrosion of Ti-6Al-4V alloy tapers. Further, it was of interest to evaluate whether use of zirconia ceramic femoral head had any effect on the fretting/crevice corrosion of the stem taper.

---

* *Ti-Nidium*™ - A proprietary process of Zimmer, Inc.

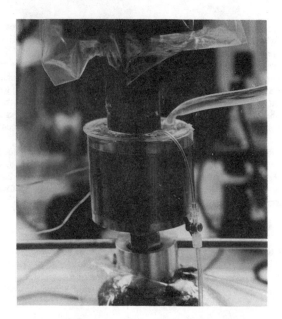

FIG. 1--Fatigue test setup showing the environmental
chamber for accelerated fretting corrosion

TABLE 1--Taper/head modular couplings investigated.

Stem Taper	Femoral Head	No. of Samples
Ti-6Al-4V	Co-Cr-Mo, Cast	5
Ti-6Al-4V	Co-Cr-Mo, Wrought	5
Ti-6Al-4V, Nitrogen Hardened Surface	Co-Cr-Mo, Wrought	5
Ti-6Al-4V, Nitrogen Hardened Surface	Zirconia Ceramic	3
Co-Cr-Mo	Co-Cr-Mo, Cast	5
Co-Cr-Mo	Co-Cr-Mo, Wrought	5
Co-Cr-Mo	Zirconia Ceramic	3

Surface Morphology Evaluation

At the completion of 10 million cycles, the femoral heads were removed from the metal tapers for evaluation of contact surfaces of both modular components. The heads and tapers were immersed in distilled water and then ultrasonically cleaned for 30 minutes. The contact surfaces were examined visually, optically, and by using a Leica S360 scanning electron microscope.

Analysis of Test Medium

The test medium was analyzed for elemental composition by atomic absorption spectroscopy. In this analysis, the debris and metal ions in the solution were digested in acid and the resultant solution was evaporated to obtain a solid residue. The elemental analysis was reported in ppm, based on the original test solution volume.

Assessment of Fretting/Corrosion Induced Changes

The condition of the taper/socket surfaces was classified into five different groups depending on the severity of fretting and/or corrosion induced changes. The measurement of these changes was made on a scale of 1-6 and various levels on this scale are described in Table 2.

TABLE 2--Evaluation of modular interfaces on a 1-6 scale.

Level	Observations
1	No Fretting, Corrosion, or Discoloration of Contact Surfaces
2	Fretting < 10% of the Contact Surface, Debris on the Contact Surfaces
3	Fretting > 10% of the Contact Surface, Debris on the Contact Surfaces
4	Chemical Etching of Structure, Fretting, Debris on the Contact Surfaces
5	Corrosion Pits and Fretting, Debris on the Contact Surfaces
6	Severe Corrosion (>50% surface area corroded), Fretting, Debris on the Contact Surfaces

RESULTS AND DISCUSSION

A large variation in the fretting/corrosion condition of the modular head/taper components of retrieved hip joints has been reported by different investigators [2-7]. Brown et al. [10] evaluated the severity of surface changes on a time scale and found a correlation for mixed metal joints. However, no differences in stem taper/head size, geometry or initial surface finish of tapers were accounted for in this analysis. Cook et al. [11] found no correlation between the corrosion and time *in vivo*. It was observed that for two hip stems retrieved after similar implantation periods, the severity of fretting/corrosion induced changes varied significantly. This study was therefore aimed to produce surface morphological changes representative of some of the most severe observations reported.

All stem tapers of modular head/taper joints tested in various material and surface condition combinations survived 10 million cycles without fracture. The surface morphology of modular interfaces of tapers and head bores for each combination studied is described in the following. The surface morphology, representative of a Ti-6Al-4V taper tested with a cast Co-Cr-Mo alloy head is shown in Figure 2. The surface morphology of the head bore surface is shown in Figure 3. The titanium alloy taper showed discoloration and debris in a region near the distal end of the contact surface. The energy dispersive x-ray (EDS) analysis of the debris showed Cr, Mo and a small peak of Co in the spectrum in addition to Ti, Al and V characteristics of the taper material. The debris on the inside surface of the bore showed high Cr and Mo peaks with small peaks of Co and Ti. The presence of Ti in these deposits suggested taper material transfer onto the head bore. Thick, plate-like, deposits on either of the contact surfaces showed "mud cracking". An etched structure showing carbides typical of a cast Co-Cr-Mo alloy was observed underneath these deposits in the bore (Fig. 4). Such etching of carbide structures has been reported by Gilbert et al. [6] on a retrieved head bore surface. The taper surface showed leaching of material in the axial direction (the micromotion direction). Preferential leaching of cobalt from the head material was also noticed (Fig. 5). The surface changes were categorized at level 4. The debris and metal ions released during fretting/corrosion fatigue testing into test media were analyzed by atomic absorption spectroscopy and the elemental analysis is shown

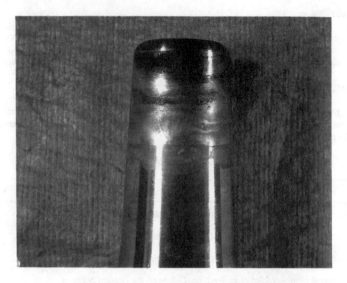

FIG. 2--The surface morphology of a Ti-6Al-4V alloy
taper tested with a cast Co-Cr-Mo alloy femoral head.

in Table 3. *Ti-Nidium* surface hardened titanium alloy tapers tested with cast Co-Cr-Mo heads released much less debris (Table 3), and showed fewer surface morphological changes (Fig. 6). While no etching of structure on taper contact surface was noticed, the head bore surface showed etched structure close to the head opening.

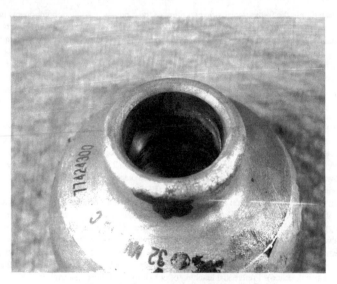

FIG. 3--Surface morphology of a cast Co-Cr-Mo
alloy head tested on a Ti-6Al-4V alloy taper.

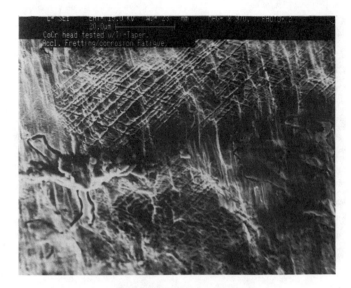

FIG. 4--Etched carbides on a cast Co-Cr-Mo
alloy head (contact surface in the bore).

In the wrought Co-Cr-Mo alloy heads coupled on either non-nitrided or nitrided titanium alloy tapers, the surface changes and the debris generated were much less evident compared to cast Co-Cr-Mo alloy tapers. On the scoring scale, the changes on the surface hardened titanium alloy taper corresponded to level 2, and the bore showed surface morphological changes corresponding to level 3. The fretting particulates and metal ions released during testing are also shown in Table 3. The modular joints of *Ti-Nidium* surface hardened Ti-6Al-4V alloy tapers and wrought Co-Cr-Mo alloy femoral heads showed a reduced effect of fretting corrosion induced surface morphological changes and the amount of debris released.

TABLE 3--Chemical composition of test media
showing the nature of debris and metal ions released.

Taper	Head	Ti ppm	Al ppm	V ppm	Co ppm	Cr ppm	Mo ppm	Zr ppm
Ti-6Al-4V	Co-Cr-Mo (Cast)	52±14	10±4	6±2	460±86	290±37	3±1.2	—
Ti-6Al-4V	Co-Cr-Mo (Wrought)	7±3	11±2	7±2	209±52	86±17	0.8±0.6	—
Ti-6Al-4V (Hardened)	Co-Cr-Mo (Cast)	8±4	8.2±2	5.6±1.6	171±24	72±10	1.3±0.3	—
Ti-6Al-4V (Hardened)	Co-Cr-Mo (Wrought)	6±1.5	1±0.4	<1.0	53±9	13±2	5±0.8	—
Co-Cr-Mo	Co-Cr-Mo (Cast)	—	—	—	38±12	3.3±0.8	0.3±0.15	—
Co-Cr-Mo	Co-Cr-Mo (Wrought)	—	—	—	5.5±1.8	1.1±0.6	0.5±0.2	—
Ti-6Al-4V (Hardened)	Zirconia	<0.5	0.1	0.1	—	—	—	<0.1
Co-Cr-Mo	Zirconia	—	—	—	<0.1	<0.1	<0.1	<0.1

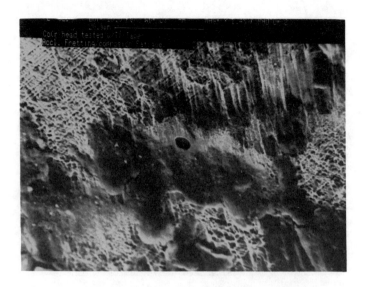

FIG. 5--Preferential leaching of a Co-Cr-Mo alloy head.

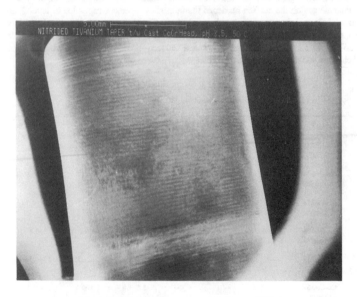

FIG. 6--Morphology changes on the nitrogen diffusion
surface hardened Ti-6Al-4V alloy taper.

The Co-Cr-Mo alloy tapers tested with cast Co-Cr-Mo alloy heads also showed surface morphological changes due to fretting corrosion (Fig. 7). The taper showed some indication of pitting on the medial side. The deposits on the taper surface showed Cr, Mo and a small Co peak in the EDS spectrum. The ratio of Co, Cr and Mo peaks in this spectrum was not characteristic of the taper material. Likewise, the deposits on the femoral head (Fig. 7) showed higher Cr and a smaller Co content compared with the base material.

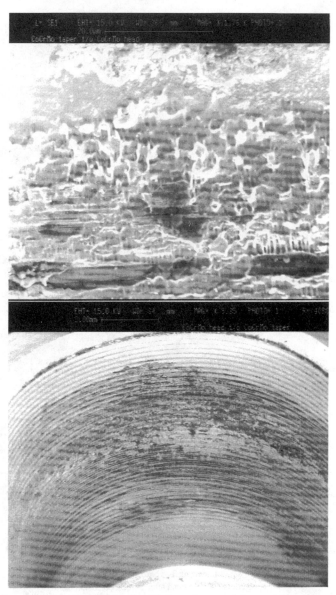

FIG. 7--Scanning electron micrographs showing the surface morphology and deposits on a Co-Cr-Mo taper and a Co-Cr-Mo head after fretting corrosion testing to 10 million cycles.

The etching of the cast structure of the femoral head was identical to that tested with a titanium taper. The debris released during testing is shown in Table 3. The wrought Co-Cr-Mo femoral heads coupled with Co-Cr-Mo tapers showed smaller amounts of debris with a chemistry identical to that observed for cast heads. In either coupling, there was no evidence of grain boundary etching on the taper surface.

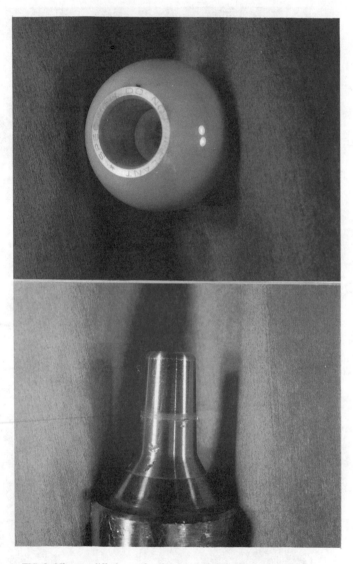

FIG. 8--Nitrogen diffusion surface hardened Ti-6Al-4V alloy taper and the zirconia ceramic head after fretting corrosion testing.

The titanium alloy and cobalt-chromium-molybdenum alloy tapers, when tested with zirconia ceramic femoral heads, showed very small amounts of fretting induced surface changes and debris (Fig. 8). The analysis of debris on the taper surface indicated a Zr peak on rarely encountered small particles. The other elemental peaks observed were characteristic of the taper material. There was no indication of corrosion on the metallic taper. The surface changes appeared to be at level 2. The zirconia ceramic bore showed discoloration (Fig. 8) which indicated elemental peaks of taper material in the EDS analysis. The surface changes in the bore corresponded to level 1. The test media appeared clear and the media analysis indicated trace amounts of elements characteristic of the taper material (Table 3).

Summarizing the results of the test media analysis, it is observed that titanium alloy and cobalt-chromium-molybdenum alloy tapers tested with cast cobalt-chromium-molybdenum had released the largest amount of debris followed by wrought Co-Cr-Mo alloy heads. Nitrogen diffusion surface hardening of the titanium alloy taper surface significantly reduced the debris generated. The zirconia ceramic femoral heads tested with either metallic taper had the minimum amounts of debris generated during fretting corrosion fatigue testing. It may be emphasized that even in the worst samples, no large quantities of particulates were released and there was no indication that any of the tested tapers were at risk of accelerated failure due to fretting/corrosion.

In all metal head/taper combinations there was consistency in the chemistry of debris observed on taper and bore surfaces. While Ti-6Al-4V tapers showed the presence of titanium in the debris, the primary constituents of debris were chromium and molybdenum indicated by their high peaks in the EDS spectrum. The similar metal joints also showed a high chromium and molybdenum content in the debris. The test media, in contrast, showed a higher cobalt content suggesting that cobalt was easily dissolved in solution. Formation of debris of this nature supports the mechanical induced chemical phenomena, proposed by Gilbert et al. [6], being operative at the joint interfaces. In this mechanism, the passivation layer breaks due to fretting and then repassivation occurs with available oxygen in the crevice. This process is repeated under cyclic loading until no more oxygen is available for repassivation, enabling the chemical phenomenon that occurs.

CONCLUSIONS

An experimental setup was developed for *in vitro* testing of modular head/taper joints to simulate the *in vivo* changes observed on the contact surfaces. A low pH Ringer's solution maintained at 50°C, used as test media, appeared to simulate the *in vivo* phenomena satisfactorily. The morphological changes on modular joints showed considerable congruence to those reported on retrieved joints. Even in the worst case studied, no large quantities of particulates were generated and there was no indication that any of the tested tapers were at risk of accelerated failure due to fretting/corrosion. It was demonstrated that nitrogen diffusion surface hardening of Ti-6Al-4V titanium alloy tapers significantly improved their resistance to fretting corrosion.

ACKNOWLEDGEMENT

The authors thank Jennifer Price, Monna Baum, and John Davis for their assistance in experimental work.

REFERENCES

[1]   McKellop, H., Gogan, W., and Ebramzadeh, E., Luck, J., and Sasmiento, A., "Metal-Metal Wear in Metal-Plastic Prosthetic Joints," Transactions of the Society for Biomaterials, Vol. XIII, 1990, pp. 144.

[2]   Collier, J. P., Surprenant, V. A., and Jensen, R. E., Transactions of the Society for Biomaterials, Vol. XIV, 1991, pp. 144.

[3]   Collier, J. P., Surprenant, V. A., Jensen, R. E., and Mayor, M. B., "Corrosion at the Interface of Cobalt-Alloy Heads on Titanium Alloy Stems," Clinical Orthopaedics, No. 271, 1991, pp. 305-312.

[4]   Collier, J. P., Surprenant, V. A., and Jensen, R. E., Mayor, M. B., and Surprenant, H. P., "Corrosion Between the Components of Modular Femoral Hip Prostheses," The Journal of Bone and Joint Surgery, Vol. 74B, No. 4, 1992, pp. 511-517.

[5]   Mathiesen, E. B., Lindgren, J. U., Biomgren, G. G. A., and Reinholt, F. P., "Corrosion of Modular Hip Prostheses," The Journal of Bone and Joint Surgery, Vol. 73B, No. 4, 1991, pp. 569-575.

[6]   Gilbert, J. L., Buckley, C. A., and Jacobs, J. J., "In Vivo corrosion of Modular Hip Prosthesis Components in Mixed and Similar Metal Combinations. The effect of crevice, stress, motion and alloy coupling." Journal of Biomedical Materials Research, Vol. 27, No. 12, 1993, pp. 1533-1544.

[7]   Jacobs, J. J., Skipore, A. K., Black, J., Urban, R. M., and Galante, J. O., "Release and Excretion of Metal in Patients," Journal of Bone and Joint Surgery, Vol. 73A, No. 10, 1991, pp. 1475-1486.

[8]   Flemming, C., Brown, S. A., and Payer, J. H., "Mechanical Testing for Fretting Corrosion of Modular Total Hip Tapers," ASTM STP 1173, Kambic, H. E., Yokobori, A. T., Eds., American Society for Testing and Materials, Philadelphia, 1994, pp. 156-166.

[9]   Bhambri, S. K., and Gilbertson, L. N., "Characterization and Quantification of Fretting Particulates Generated in Ceramic/Metal and Metal/Metal Modular Head/Taper System," ASTM STP 1173, Kambic, H. E., Yokobori, A. T., Eds., American Society for Testing and Materials, Philadelphia, 1994, pp. 111-126.

[10]   Brown, S. A., Flemming, C. A. C., and Kawalec, J. S., et al., "Fretting Corrosion Accelerates Crevice Corrosion of Modular Hip Tapers," Journal of Applied Biomaterials, Vol. 6, No. 1, 1995, pp. 19-26.

[11]   Cook, S. D., Barrack, R. L., and Clemow, A. J. T., "Corrosion and Wear at the Modular Interface of Uncemented Femoral Stems," The Journal of Bone and Joint Surgery, Vol. 76B, No. 1, 1994, pp. 68-72.

Jay R. Goldberg[1], Christine A. Buckley[2], Joshua J. Jacobs[3], and Jeremy L. Gilbert[1]

CORROSION TESTING OF MODULAR HIP IMPLANTS

REFERENCE: Goldberg, J. R., Buckley, C. A., Jacobs, J. J., and Gilbert, J. L., "**Corrosion Testing of Modular Hip Implants,**" *Modularity of Orthopedic Implants, ASTM STP 1301,* Donald E. Marlowe, Jack E. Parr, and Michael B. Mayor, Eds., American Society for Testing and Materials, 1997.

ABSTRACT: Flexibility in sizing, lower inventory requirements, and the ability to choose materials with optimum physical properties for each component have made modular hip implants the design of choice for most orthopedic surgeons. However, the presence of surface asperities and angular mismatch between the head and neck components can result in the formation of a crevice between the taper surfaces of the assembled couple. This crevice may be large enough to allow fluid ingress and fretting to occur which can lead to crevice and fretting corrosion.

    This paper describes several test methods used to duplicate the fretting behavior of modular taper components and determine the electrochemical changes that occur as the result of fretting corrosion. Mixed and similar metal modular taper junctions were tested in phosphate buffered saline solution with and without the application of a cyclic load. Fretting currents, open circuit potential (OCP), and pH, pO_2, and [Cl-] of solution trapped inside the spaces between the head and neck components were measured. Metal ion concentrations in fluid trapped inside similar metal taper junctions were measured. The effects of load magnitude on OCP and fretting currents were determined. Test components and trapped solution were inspected and analyzed for signs of corrosion. Results of testing support a hypothesis of mechanically assisted crevice corrosion and are presented.

KEYWORDS: corrosion, fretting, crevice, implants, modularity, debris, oxide films, metal ions, cobalt-chrome alloy, titanium alloy.

---

[1]Research Fellow and Associate Professor, respectively, Division of Biological Materials, Northwestern University, Chicago, IL 60611.

[2]Assistant Professor, Department of Mechanical Engineering, Rose-Hulman Institute of Technology, Terre Haute, IN 47803.

[3]Associate Professor, Department of Orthopedic Surgery, Rush Presbyterian-St. Luke's Medical Center, Chicago, IL 60612.

INTRODUCTION

Modular total hip prostheses are preferred by many orthopedic surgeons for use in total hip arthroplasties. There are three major benefits to using these implants. First, they allow the surgeon to choose the appropriate neck length and head diameter at the time of surgery, facilitating more precise joint reconstruction. Second, they provide a choice of head and neck materials, allowing the surgeon to take advantage of the low stiffness and high fatigue resistance offered by a Ti-6Al-4V stem, and the high wear resistance provided by a Co-Cr-Mo head. Third, greater flexibility in sizing can be provided by maintaining a set of head and neck components of various diameters in the hospital inventory. Less inventory would be required than if all sizes of traditional single component hip implants were kept on hand, resulting in lower inventory costs to the hospital.

Problems with Modular Hip Implants

The head and neck components of modular hip implants are manufactured to tolerances that can result in the formation of a gap between the two mating surfaces at the taper interface. This gap may be large enough to allow fluid to enter and remain stagnant, and may allow small scale movement (fretting) of the head relative to the neck during cyclic loading. These conditions are conducive to crevice and fretting corrosion, respectively. In-vivo corrosion in the tapered interfaces of similar (Co-Cr-Mo neck/Co-Cr-Mo head) and mixed metal (Ti-6Al-4V neck/Co-Cr-Mo head) modular hip components has been reported [1-6].

Corrosion can lead to mechanical failure and metal debris generation. Gilbert, et. al. [7], reported on two modular hip implants that fractured in the neck close to the head/neck junction due to intergranular corrosion fatigue failure. This resulted from a combination of intergranular corrosive attack initiating at the neck taper surface and cyclic loading. Particulate and soluble metal debris have been recovered from periprosthetic tissues and metal ions have been found in various body organs of patients with modular hip implants [8]. Jacobs, et. al. [9], reported elevated serum cobalt and urine chromium concentrations as a function of the degree of corrosion at the taper interface and suggested that fretting corrosion may be a dominant mechanism of metal release in patients with modular hip implants. Fretting can disrupt the passive oxide layers present on the surfaces of Co-Cr-Mo and Ti-6Al-4V alloys and produce metal oxide particles. These particles can become trapped between the taper surfaces and result in third body wear, accelerating wear and fretting corrosion.

Corrosion products can produce a variety of biological effects. Urban, et. al. [10], studied the migration of solid corrosion products from the modular head/neck junction to the periprosthetic tissues, and concluded that corrosion products may indirectly contribute to bone resorption, osteolysis, and loosening of the implant. Svensson, et. al. [11], reported on a patient that developed a pseudotumor close to a Co-Cr-Mo modular hip implant. They concluded that the pseudotumor was due to a hypersensitivity or allergic reaction to corrosion products triggered by the local release of metal ions resulting from crevice corrosion.

Retrieval Analyses

Several retrieval analyses of modular hip implants have been performed. Various results have been reported and there is disagreement on the types of corrosion observed. Several hypotheses have been presented to explain these observations. Lieberman, et. al. [1], reported that fretting and crevice corrosion were observed on the taper surfaces of two of ten (20%) retrieved mixed metal implants, and no corrosion was observed in twenty-six similar metal implants, or twelve press fit, silicone sealed, mixed metal implants. The authors hypothesized that micromotion and trapped fluid are precursors to damage and corrosion at the taper interface.

Cook, et. al. [6], reported wear and corrosion in 7% of the similar metal and 34.5% of the mixed metal implants evaluated. These characteristics were consistently observed at the distal portion of the taper interface where there was high stress and access to fluid. The authors reported that the damage observed in the retrieved implants was consistent with that of a combination of fretting, crevice, and galvanic corrosion, and hypothesized that fretting led to a breach in the passive layers of the alloy surfaces which was followed by a combination of crevice and galvanic corrosion.

Collier, et. al. have cited several studies in support of the hypothesis that corrosion observed in modular hip implants is accelerated by galvanic corrosion [3-5]. In one study they reported corrosion in 52% of the mixed metal implants and none of the similar metal implants evaluated. No fretting was observed on any of the implants and scanning electron microscopy (SEM) of corroded areas showed deep pits characteristic of corrosion with no indications of fretting.

In a study of one hundred forty-eight retrieved implants, Gilbert, et. al. [12], reported that fretting and corrosion were observed in both mixed and similar metal implants. This was attributed to a complex mechanically assisted crevice corrosion process initiated by the disruption of the oxide layer on one or both of the components. In this process, crevice conditions created by taper geometry and mechanical factors such as wear (fretting) or stress accelerated corrosion.

Previous Work

Several studies have been conducted to investigate the effects of mechanical loading on fretting and corrosion of modular hip prostheses and have yielded different results. In a study involving short duration, cyclic loading of similar and mixed metal head/neck taper assemblies, no measurable fretting debris or evidence of fretting was observed, suggesting that long term in-vivo fretting corrosion should not occur with either material couple [13]. Another study of cyclically loaded mixed metal modular hip prostheses included measurement of fretting currents and suggested that fretting does occur at the head/neck interface and may be a factor in the corrosion observed in the taper interfaces of retrieved modular implants [14]. Others have suggested that corrosion at the head/neck interface is initiated by fretting and repassivation of the metal within the taper crevice that can lead to crevice corrosion [15].

Finally, studies involving measurements of fretting currents, open circuit potential (OCP), and electrochemical indicators of crevice corrosion such as pH, chloride ion concentration ([Cl-]), and pO_2 have been conducted [16, 17]. These studies support the hypothesis of mechanically assisted crevice corrosion.

Mechanically Assisted Crevice Corrosion

The corrosion observed in the Morse taper region of modular hip implants has been attributed to the presence of a gap between the taper surfaces. This gap (crevice) allows fluid to enter, and during cyclic loading, allows the two surfaces to slide against each other (fretting). The interactive effects of taper geometry, fluid ingress, and mechanical loading on modular taper corrosion have been hypothesized in a model of mechanically assisted crevice corrosion (MACC), proposed by Gilbert, et. al. [12]. This model is summarized in Figure 1. The initial crevice geometry is created by the fit between the head and neck components. Physiological fluids penetrate into the crevice. A mechanical event such as stress or fretting due to external loading of the implant results in fracture of the passive oxide layer present on the taper surfaces. The exposed reactive base metal repassivates, consuming solution dissolved oxygen, hydrolyzing water, and releasing metal ions. As fretting or stress cycling continue due to cyclic loading of the hip implant (as in walking), the fracture/repassivation process continues, resulting in the depletion of dissolved oxygen in the solution present in the crevice between the head and neck. This leads to an excess of metal ions in solution and results in the rapid penetration of chloride ions into the crevice to react with the metal ions and maintain charge neutrality. The metal chlorides can hydrolyze water to form metal hydroxides and hydrochloric acid (HCl). Continuation of the fracture/repassivation process decreases the pH of the crevice solution and autocatalyzes the corrosion process until the oxide film becomes thermodynamically unstable and active corrosion occurs. The processes associated with crevice corrosion can occur in the absence of fretting but at a much lower rate.

Drops in open circuit potential (OCP) between the head and neck components due to in-vitro cyclic loading of modular tapers have been reported [16, 17]. If the OCP is reduced to a level within the active-passive transition region for the oxide, the oxide will become less stable and less able to reform after fracture. However, OCP will still be high enough for corrosion to continue. Decreases in OCP and pH can accelerate active corrosion of the base metal.

Study Objectives

The oxide fracture/repassivation process occurring within the taper crevice and electrochemical changes in the solution inside the head are central to the MACC model. In order to better understand the mechanisms leading to taper crevice corrosion, knowledge of the mechanical and electrochemical interactions present within the modular taper is important. This knowledge could help determine which design modifications might be helpful in reducing or eliminating modular taper corrosion and its associated problems.

The objectives of this paper are to describe and present the results of an in-vitro fretting corrosion test used to investigate mechanically assisted crevice corrosion of

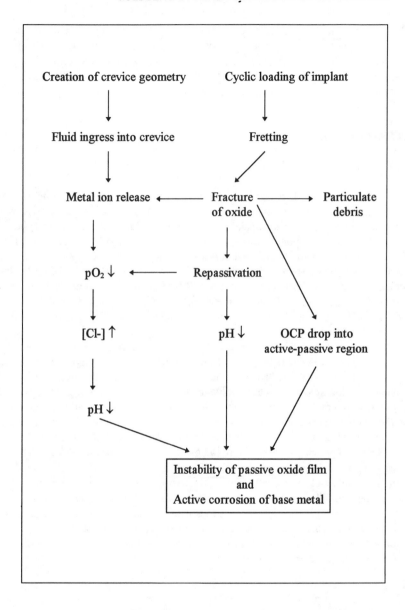

FIG. 1--Proposed model of mechanically assisted crevice corrosion (MACC).

similar and mixed metal modular tapers. The effects of load magnitude and number of load cycles on fretting currents and OCP will be presented, in addition to the changes in crevice solution chemistry (pH, [Cl-], and pO_2) resulting when mechanical loads are absent and present. Differences observed between mixed and similar metal couples will be discussed.

MATERIALS AND METHODS

Sample Preparation

Three mixed and three similar metal modular taper junctions were produced using the same manufacturing processes and specifications (surface finish, taper tolerances, etc.) as those used to produce commercially available modular hip implants (Zimmer, Inc. Warsaw, IN). Head components were made of Co-Cr-Mo (ASTM Standard Specification for Cast Cobalt-Chromium-Molybdenum Alloy for Surgical Implant Applications (F-75)). Neck tapers were machined from Co-Cr-Mo and Ti-6Al-4V (ASTM Standard Specification for Wrought Titanium 6A 1-4V ELI Alloy for Surgical Implant Applications (F-136)). Components used in similar metal taper junctions were passivated per ASTM Standard Practice for Surface Preparation and Marking of Metallic Surgical Implants (F-86) prior to assembly.

Oxygen, pH, and chloride specific electrodes were inserted into the space between the proximal head and neck taper surfaces through holes drilled through the top of the head. The holes were then sealed with silicone. Heads used in two similar metal couples contained a second hole with a check valve to allow for intermittent insertion of the pH electrode with internal reference and provide adequate sealing of the interior head space when the electrode was not in the head. This was done to minimize changes in solution chemistry of the fluid trapped inside the head due to the presence of the electrode.

Neck components were bolted to the base of a corrosion test cell with the neck situated at a 35° angle to the vertical. A wire used to monitor OCP was connected to the bolt and neck base and sealed with silicone. A plastic bag was sealed around the base of the neck taper and filled with phosphate buffered saline (PBS) solution to a level just above the external taper junction in order to isolate all other potential fretting interfaces from the solution. This ensured that only currents resulting from fretting at the head/neck junction would be detected. The head was then immersed in and filled with the PBS solution, and firmly assembled onto the neck.

Test Set-Up

The corrosion test cell containing the assembled taper junction is shown in Figure 2. OCP was monitored with a high impedance voltmeter (EG&G Princeton Applied Research, Model 362 Scanning Potentiostat, Princeton, NJ) connected to the neck component and a saturated calomel electrode (SCE) as a reference. Fretting currents were measured with a zero resistance ammeter (Keithley, Model 485 Autoranging Picoammeter, Cleveland, OH) connected to the neck component and a Ti-6Al-4V rod as a

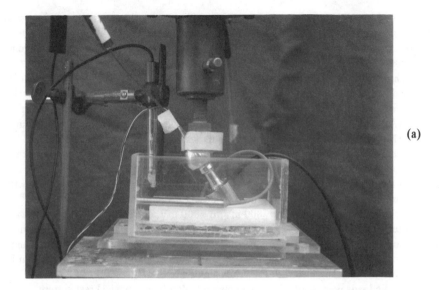

(a)

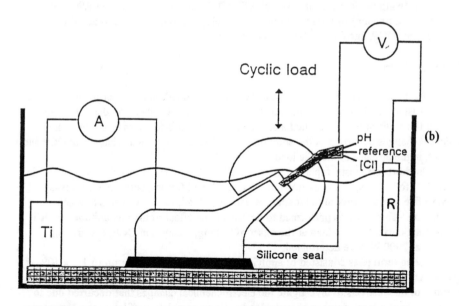

(b)

FIG. 2--(a) Corrosion test cell containing the assembled taper junction and various electrodes. The plastic bag and PBS solution are not shown. (b) Schematic of the test set-up.

counter electrode. This electrode configuration differed from that used in a previous study [17], and allowed independent and simultaneous measurement of OCP and fretting currents without the need to impose an external potential, which could effect any ongoing corrosion processes.

Three different electrodes were used to monitor pH, [Cl-], and pO_2 of the solution inside the head. A pH reference microelectrode (LAZAR, Model PH146-U, Los Angeles, CA) with a self-contained reference electrode was used to monitor pH. A silver/silver chloride (Ag/AgCl) electrode made from silver metal wire chlorided in saturated sodium chloride (NaCl) solution at +1.0 V for two hours was used with the pH reference to monitor chloride ion concentration. Chloride and pH electrodes were calibrated prior to insertion into the head.

A set of platinum wires was used to measure changes in pO_2. Cyclic voltammetry was performed with the two wires acting as working and counter electrodes. As the working electrode was cycled from -800 mV to +800 mV, current flowing between it and the counter electrode was measured. When testing similar metal taper junctions, the neck component was used as the counter electrode. Cyclic voltammograms were plotted and currents at -800 mV were used as a measure of the amount of oxygen available in solution to react with the working electrode, and thus a measure of pO_2.

Cyclic loads were applied using an electrohydraulic mechanical test system (Instron, Model 1350, Canton, MA). A computer data acquisition system consisting of an A/D board (National Instruments, Model ATMIO16, Austin, TX), and LabWindows® (National Instruments) software, was used to develop custom software to acquire and analyze load, OCP, current, pH, [Cl-], and pO_2 data.

<u>Test Procedures</u>

Rest, short term, and long term tests were performed on the taper junctions. Rest tests consisted of allowing the taper junction to sit in the PBS filled corrosion test cell without the application of a cyclic load. The purpose of this test was to monitor the chemical changes occurring in the solution inside the head, as well as changes in OCP and current, in the absence of a cyclic load.

In short term tests, taper junctions were loaded at 5 Hz, at maximum cyclic loads from 50 N to 2000 N, and back down to 0 N. OCP and fretting currents were measured three to five minutes after initial loading at each new load, to allow values to reach equilibrium. This test was performed to determine the effect of load magnitude on OCP and fretting currents. The load at the onset of fretting, changes in OCP, and fretting currents at 2000 N were determined.

Long term tests consisted of applying a 2000 N, 5 Hz load for up to 1.3×10^6 cycles: OCP, fretting currents, pH, [Cl-], and pO_2 were measured periodically. The purpose of this test was to investigate the electrochemical changes that occurred due to the presence of a large number of cyclic loads. Upon completion of long term tests, taper components were visually inspected for signs of corrosion. SEM was used to evaluate taper surfaces. Fluid trapped inside the heads was removed and visually inspected.

The saline solution trapped between the head and neck components of similar metal tapers was collected. Inductively Coupled Plasma Atomic Emission Spectroscopy

(ICPAES) was used to detect and quantify the concentration of Co, Cr, and Mo ions present in these fluid samples. Fluid was collected from unloaded as well as loaded samples. This analysis was done to investigate the effect of loading on the generation of metal ions.

Statistical analyses were performed on pH, [Cl-], OCP, and fretting current data. Analysis of variance (ANOVA) and Newman-Keuls post-hoc tests were used to determine if there were any statistically significant differences in these dependent variables between mixed and similar metal samples.

RESULTS

Rest Tests

Results from rest tests are summarized in Table 1. Decreases in pH and pO_2, and increases in [Cl-] were observed, to varying degrees, with all samples tested. Changes in pH and [Cl-] were larger with mixed metal couples. However, no statistically significant differences in these variables were found between similar and mixed metal couples.

TABLE 1--Summary of rest test results for mixed and similar metal tapers.

Sample	Duration (hrs)	ΔpH (units) (Initial pH~7.0)	Δ[Cl-] (M)	$\Delta pO_2/pO_{2initial}$ x 100%
Mixed Metal:				
1	65	-3	+1.8	...
2	25	-1	+0.4	-45%
3	48	-3	+0.15	...
Similar Metal:				
1	145	-1	+0.87	...
2	116	-1.5	+0.4	-54%
3	142	-1.7	+1.0	...

Three cyclic voltammograms recorded at 0, 18, and 116 hours are shown in Figure 3 for a similar metal couple. The decreases in current measured at -800 mV indicate a decrease in the amount of oxygen dissolved in the solution inside the head. Similar decreases in pO_2 were observed with mixed and similar metal couples. Differences in the magnitude of changes in this current for each sample are affected by differences in surface areas of the platinum wires exposed to solution. To eliminate this surface area effect, percent changes in initial pO_2 values are reported in Table 1.

Fretting current and OCP behaved similarly with both types of tapers. Fretting current started slightly positive immediately after assembly of the head/neck junction and quickly reached a steady state value close to zero. OCP began very negative after assembly and reached an equilibrium value close to zero at the end of the test.

<u>Short Term Tests</u>

Results from short term tests are summarized in Table 2. Observed changes in OCP, mean fretting currents, and fretting current amplitudes were similar for all tapers tested. Initial OCP values were between 0 and -100 mV and began to decrease at loads as low as 100 N (mixed metal) and 130 N (similar metal). OCP typically dropped to about -350 mV at a load of 2000 N, as shown in Figure 4a. Mean fretting currents and fretting current amplitudes increased with increasing loads as shown in Figures 4b and 4c. The point where the slope of the mean fretting current curve significantly changes indicates the load at the onset of fretting (and the onset of fretting currents). This load ranged from 250 to 600 N for mixed metal and 400 to 1320 N for similar metal tapers and was higher for samples that were seated with an initial 2000 N static load prior to testing.

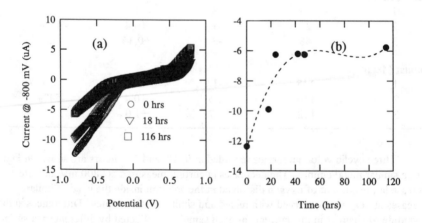

FIG. 3--(a) Cyclic voltammograms made at 0, 18, and 116 hours. Note the decrease in current measured at a potential of -800 mV indicating a decrease in oxygen dissolved in the PBS inside the head. (b) Plot of current measured at a potential of -800 mV vs. time.

TABLE 2--Summary of short term test results for mixed and similar metal tapers.

Sample	ΔOCP (mV) @ 2000 N	Load at onset of $I_{fretting}$ (N)	I_{amp} (μA) (peak to peak) @ 2000 N	I_{mean} (μA) @ 2000 N
Mixed Metal:				
1	-200	450	...	...
2	-210	250	0.84	0.45
3	-250	600	1.35	1.45
Similar Metal:				
1	-360	440	0.94	0.58
2	-225	400	0.25	0.27
3	-140	1320	0.68	0.41

As load was decreased, OCP increased to about 100 mV below the initial OCP for the particular test. Mean fretting currents and fretting current amplitudes typically decreased back to their initial values. Hysteresis between loading and unloading curves was observed with OCP recovering more slowly than fretting currents. Less hysteresis was observed in a mixed metal taper that was seated with an initial 2000 N static load. No statistically significant differences were found in short term test results between mixed and similar metal couples.

Long Term Tests

Results of long term tests are summarized in Table 3. Changes observed in OCP, mean fretting currents, pH, [Cl-], and pO_2 were similar for all samples tested, and were similar to some of the results observed in rest tests. Figure 5 shows the results of a 90 hour rest test immediately followed by a long term test. The central vertical line indicates the point where cyclic loading of the mixed metal taper began. Initiation of cyclic loading resulted in an increase in mean fretting current and a 200 mV drop in OCP. As loading continued, mean fretting current and OCP tended to drift back to equilibrium values close to 0 μA and 0 mV, respectively.

Decreases in pH and pO_2, and increases in [Cl-] were observed as cyclic loading continued. In one mixed metal sample no change in pH was observed. The abrupt change in mean current and OCP seen at 750,000 cycles in Figure 5 may have been due to a sudden movement of the head on the neck. The resulting response was similar to that observed at the onset of loading. A slight decrease in [Cl-] and increase in pH were observed at the onset of loading. This may have been the result of pumping of fresh PBS into and stagnant PBS out of the inside of the head as it became firmly seated on the neck. No statistically significant differences in long term test results were found between mixed and similar metal couples.

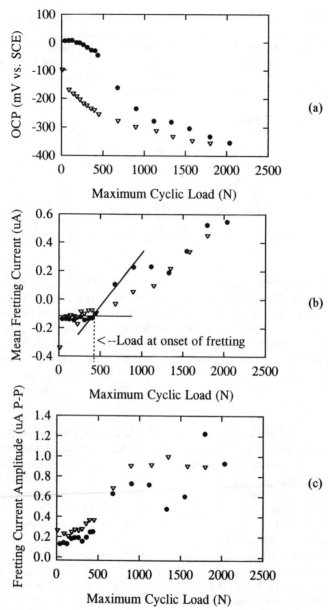

FIG. 4--(a) OCP, (b) mean fretting current, and (c) fretting current amplitude versus maximum cyclic load for a short term test of a similar metal taper. Closed circles and open triangles represent loading and unloading curves, respectively. Note hysteresis in curves. Load at onset of fretting is determined by finding value of load where slope of fretting current curve changes significantly and is shown in (b). OCP and fretting current amplitude also begin to change significantly near this value (440 N).

TABLE 3--Summary of long term test data for mixed and similar metal tapers.

Sample	Duration (cycles)	ΔpH (pH units)	$\Delta[Cl-]$ (M)	I_{mean} @ 100K cycles (μA)	I_{mean} @ 600K cycles (μA)	$\Delta pO_2/$ $pO_{2initial}$ x 100%
Mixed Metal:						
1	900,000	-1.5	+0.5	1.2	0.6	...
2	1,300,000	-2	+1.1	0.1	-0.05	...
3	1,300,000	0	+1.5	0.75	0.25	-25%
Similar Metal:						
1	950,000	-1	+1.1	0.1	0.25	-55%
2	750,000	-0.6	+2.6	0.05	0.15	-54%
3	333,000	0	+0.7	-0.03	...	...

Figure 6 is an SEM micrograph of the inside of the head of one of the mixed metal samples tested for 900,000 cycles (sample #1). The pitting and fretting corrosion seen in the micrograph is similar to that observed in retrieved implants. The OCP of this particular sample remained at between -300 and -450 mV (within the active-passive transition region) for almost the entire test instead of equilibrating back to 0 mV as the other two samples did, and may have contributed to the observed corrosion.

Inspection of similar metal taper sample #2 revealed discoloration around the neck at the distal head/neck junction after 750,000 cycles. After 950,000 cycles, a green tinted fluid was removed from the space inside the head of sample #1. Visible particulate debris was observed in the recovered fluid. After a period of a few days, the green color disappeared and the fluid become clear.

The results of ICPAES analysis of metal ion concentrations in fluid trapped between the head and neck components of similar metal tapers are summarized in Table 4. Although sample sizes are too small to make conclusions regarding the effects of loading on the generation of metal ions, the data suggests the possibility of several general trends. First, metal ions were present in the taper crevice. Second, it appears that greater quantities of metal ions were released when cyclic loads were applied. Third, the highest concentration of metal ions were detected in sample #1, which was loaded for 950,000 cycles, and contained a green tinted fluid in the space between the head and neck.

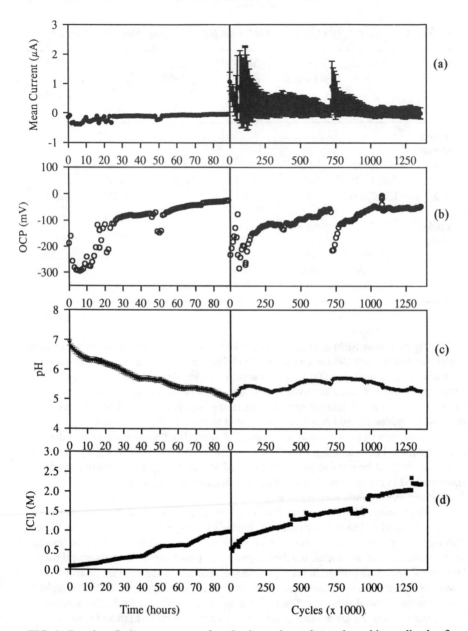

FIG. 5--Results of a long term test of a mixed metal couple conducted immediately after the completion of a 90 hour rest test. Fretting currents (a), OCP (b), pH (c), and [Cl-] (d) are plotted as a function of time to the left of the central vertical line and as a function of the number of load cycles to the right of this line.

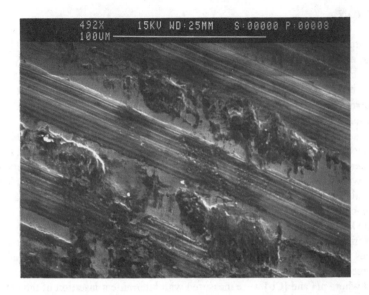

FIG. 6--Scanning electron micrograph taken inside the Co-Cr-Mo head of one of the mixed metal samples after 900,000 cycles. Evidence of pitting is much like that seen in retrieved implants.

TABLE 4--Summary of ICPAES results for similar metal tapers.

	Sample	Duration	Ionic Concentrations (ppb)		
			Cr	Co	Mo
Unloaded:	1	142 hrs	*	*	*
	2	336 hrs	*	854	*
Loaded:	1	950,000 cycles	◆	2036	244
	2	750,000 cycles	*	440	*
	3	333,000 cycles	◆	688	◆

(◆) = concentration was below detection limit,
(*) = concentration was above detection limit but below quantitation limit.

DISCUSSION

In studies of crevices between titanium electrodes and polytetrafluoroethylene discs, Yao, et. al. [18], found that the onset of crevice corrosion was indicated by a decrease in crevice solution pH, an increase in corrosion current, and a cathodic excursion in potential inside the crevice. In experiments conducted for 100 hours, no onset of crevice corrosion was observed for samples in solution less than 85°C or chloride concentration less than 1.0 M.

No sudden decrease in OCP or increase in current were observed in rest tests and visual inspection of test samples showed no visible signs of corrosion. However, the solution chemistry changes typically associated with crevice corrosion were observed, and metal ions were detected in the solution trapped between the head and neck of unloaded similar metal samples. This suggests that crevice corrosion may be occurring at a low rate in the absence of loading.

The larger changes in [Cl-] and pH observed with mixed metal tapers may be due to the specific material combination of these couples or the procedure used to monitor these values. The pH electrode, filled with saturated KCl, was sealed into the head during tests of mixed metal tapers. Prior to testing the similar metal couples, tests were conducted where pH and [Cl-] were measured with intermittent insertion of the pH electrode into the head through a port. These tests suggested that part of the increase in [Cl-] observed may have been due to leaching of KCl into the solution in the head from the electrode itself. Intermittent insertion of the pH electrode was used during testing of the similar metal tapers to eliminate this effect. It is important to note that even with this change in procedure pH and [Cl-] changes were still observed. This suggests that the observed changes in pH and [Cl-] are caused by factors other than the presence of the pH electrode.

Results of the short term tests indicate that OCP decreases, and mean fretting currents and fretting current amplitudes increase with increasing load. Significant fretting currents begin to appear at loads well below those occurring during physical activities such as walking. In one case, the application of a seating static load to the taper assembly prior to testing resulted in a slight decrease in hysteresis between loading and unloading curves and an increase in the load at the onset of fretting. This suggests that proper seating of the head onto the neck may help reduce fretting between the two components and increase the load required to initiate fretting. The load at the onset of fretting indicates the load required to initiate fracture of the oxide on the taper surface of one or both of the components and may provide a measure of fretting corrosion resistance of the oxide. Variations in this load may be due to differences in taper geometry which may control the degree of fretting. No statistically significant difference was found between loads at the onset of fretting for mixed and similar metal tapers.

Oxide fracture and repassivation occur as the result of fretting. This process results in the generation of metal ions and free electrons which produce fretting currents. Therefore, mean fretting currents and fretting current amplitudes are indications of the amount of debris, both particulate and ionic, generated by fretting. When cyclic loads were applied to the test samples, a sudden drop in OCP and increase in current was observed, indicating the onset of fretting and fretting currents. SEM analysis of a head from one of the taper samples tested showed signs of fretting and pitting corrosion. Higher concentrations of metal ions were found in the fluid trapped between the head and neck of similar metal samples that had been loaded compared to those that were not loaded. These results suggest that taper crevice corrosion is accelerated by mechanical loads.

A fluid filled taper crevice was created by the mating of the head and neck components. Cyclic loads produced fretting which caused the oxide to fracture. Subsequent repassivation produced fretting currents. Chloride concentration increased and pH and pO_2 decreased. Cyclic loads produced cathodic excursions in OCP, which dropped OCP into the active-passive transition region where the oxide is less stable and corrosion is accelerated. Higher metal ion concentrations were detected in the fluid trapped inside loaded similar metal tapers. These observations are predicted by and support our model of mechanically assisted crevice corrosion.

In general, no significant differences were found between mixed and similar metal tapers tested in this study. Differences in results may be due to variations in taper geometry between samples or changes in test procedures.

In a recent study of fretting damage between bone plates and screws, Kawalec, et. al. [22], showed that Ti-6Al-4V exhibited the greatest amount of fretting damage when fretted against itself. Damage observed between wrought Co-Cr-Mo and Ti-6Al-4V was considerably elevated. The least amount of damage was observed when Co-Cr-Mo was fretted against itself. This suggests that Co-Cr-Mo alloy may be more resistant to fretting and thus more resistant to fretting corrosion. This is further supported by scratch test measurements of oxide films of Ti-6Al-4V and Co-Cr-Mo alloys performed in our laboratory [23, 24]. Although no significant differences were observed in the short and long term tests previously discussed, differences in the incidence of corrosion seen with retrieved implants may be due to differences in the mechanical properties of the surface oxides of the two alloys and not due to galvanism. Additional samples need to be tested in order to determine if any differences or trends exist and if material combination has an effect on taper crevice corrosion.

CONCLUSIONS

The results of this study support the hypothesis of mechanically assisted crevice corrosion. Changes in solution chemistry occur, including changes in metal ion concentrations, that suggest that taper crevice corrosion may be occurring in the absence of mechanical loading. At the onset of loading, drops in OCP and increases in mean fretting currents and fretting current amplitudes indicate the initiation of fretting and fretting corrosion. OCP decreases, and mean fretting current and fretting current amplitude increase as load increases. Loads at the onset of fretting may be indicators of fretting and fretting corrosion resistance and occur at loads well below those observed during normal physical activity. Proper seating of the head onto the neck may increase the load required to fracture the oxide on the surface of either component and may reduce fretting currents and the release of metal ions and debris associated with the oxide fracture and repassivation process.

Evidence of fretting and crevice corrosion, similar to that observed in-vivo, has been observed in sample tapers tested per the test methods presented here. These methods provide a detailed and quantitative procedure for assessing the susceptibility of modular tapers to mechanically assisted crevice corrosion. The threshold cyclic load at which taper fretting currents are detected may be an indicator of the resistance of the taper oxide films to fretting and thus may be used as a measure of their resistance to modular taper corrosion. Measurement of fretting currents provides an indication of the degree of metal ion and particulate debris generation that may be expected with a particular taper design. The test methods presented here can be used to predict the effect of design variables such as material combination, taper geometry, surface characteristics, and surface modifications on fretting and crevice corrosion. These test methods will help in understanding the nature of the oxide fracture and repassivation process occurring in modular taper crevices and will help in reducing or eliminating taper crevice corrosion in modular hip implants.

This study has provided some evidence in support of our proposed model of mechanically assisted crevice corrosion. However, additional studies are needed to clearly demonstrate the nature and magnitude of the changes that have been hypothesized to occur.

Acknowledgments

The authors would like to thank Zimmer, Inc., for providing modular taper connections for testing, and Rush Medical College (NIH AR39310) and the U. S. Department of Education (NIDRR H133P0016-94) for their financial support of this work.

REFERENCES

[1]   Lieberman, J. R., Rimnac, C. M., Garvin, K. L., Klein, R. W., and Salvati, E. A., "An Analysis of the Head-Neck Taper Interface in Retrieved Hip Prostheses," Clinical Orthopedics and Related Research, Vol. 300, March 1994, pp 162-167.

[2]   Mathiesen, E. B., Lindgren, J. U., Blomgren, G. G. A., Reinholt, F. P., "Corrosion of Modular Hip Prostheses," Journal of Bone and Joint Surgery, Vol. 73-B, July 1991, pp 569-575.

[3]   Collier, J. P., Mayor, M. B., Jensen, R. E., Surprenant, V. A., Surprenant, H. E., McNamara, J. L., and Belec, L., "Mechanisms of Failure of Modular Prostheses," Clinical Orthopedics and Related Research, Vol. 285, December 1992, pp 129-139.

[4]   Collier, J. P., Surprenant, V. A., Jensen, R. E., and Mayor, M. B., "Corrosion at the Interface of Cobalt Alloy Heads on Titanium Alloy Stems," Clinical Orthopedics and Related Research, Vol. 271, October 1991, pp 305-312.

[5]   Collier, J. P., Surprenant, V. A., Jensen, R. E., Mayor, M. B., and Surprenant, H. E., "Corrosion Between the Components of Modular Femoral Hip Prostheses," Journal of Bone and Joint Surgery, Vol. 74-B, July 1992, pp 511-517.

[6]   Cook, S. D., Barrack, R. L., and Clemow, A. J. T., "Corrosion and Wear at the
        Modular Interface of Uncemented Femoral Stems," Journal of Bone and Joint
        Surgery, Vol. 76-B, January 1994, pp 68-72.
[7]   Gilbert, J. L., Buckley, C. A., Jacobs, J. J., Bertin, K. C., and Zernich, M. R.,
        "Intergranular Corrosion-Fatigue Failure of Cobalt-Alloy Femoral Stems," Journal
        of Bone and Joint Surgery, Vol. 76-A, January 1994, pp 110-115.
[8]   Michel, R., Nolte, M., Reich, M., and Loer, F., "Systemic Effects of Implanted
        Prostheses Made of Cobalt-Chromium Alloys," Archives of Orthopedic and
        Trauma Surgery, Vol. 110, 1991, pp 61-74.
[9]   Jacobs, J. J., Urban, R. M., Gilbert, J. L., Skipor, A. K., Block, J., Jasty, M., and
        Galante, J. O., "Local and Distant Products from Modularity," Clinical
        Orthopedics, Vol. 319, 1995, pp 94-105.
[10]   Urban, R. M., Jacobs, J. J., Gilbert, J. L., and Galante, J. O., "Migration of
        Corrosion Products from Modular Hip Prostheses, Particle Microanalysis and
        Histopathological Findings," Journal of Bone and Joint Surgery, Vol. 76-A,
        September 1994, pp 1345-1359.
[11]   Svensson, O., Mathiesen, E. B., Reinholt, F. P., and Blomgren, G., "Formation of
        a Fulminant Soft-Tissue Pseudotumor after Uncemented Hip Arthroplasty,"
        Journal of Bone and Joint Surgery, Vol. 70-A, September 1988, pp 1238-1242.
[12]   Gilbert, J. L., Buckley, C. A., and Jacobs, J. J., "In-vivo Corrosion of Modular Hip
        Prosthesis Components in Mixed and Similar Metal Combinations. The Effect of
        Crevice, Stress, Motion, and Alloy Coupling," Journal of Biomedical Materials
        Research, Vol. 27, 1993, pp 1533-1544.
[13]   Fricker, D. C., and Shivanath, R., "Fretting Corrosion Studies of Universal
        Femoral Head Prostheses and Cone Taper Spigots," Biomaterials, Vol. 11,
        September 1990, pp 495-500.
[14]   Fleming, C. A. C., Brown, S. A., and Payer, J. H., "Mechanical Testing for
        Fretting Corrosion of Modular Total Hip Tapers," Biomaterials Mechanical
        Properties, ASTM STP 1173, H. E. Kambic and A. T. Tokobori, Jr., Eds.,
        American Society for Testing and Materials, Philadelphia, 1994, pp 156-166.
[15]   Brown, S. A., et. al., "Fretting Corrosion Testing of Modular Hip Designs,"
        Fourth World Biomaterials Conference, 1992, pg. 268.
[16]   Gilbert, J. L., Buckley, C. A., Jacobs, J. J., and Lautenschlager, E. P., "In-vitro
        Mechanical-Electrochemical Testing of the Fretting Corrosion Process in Modular
        Femoral Tapers," Transactions of the 41st Annual Meeting of the Orthopedic
        Research Society, The Orthopedic Research Society, Palatine, IL, Vol. 20, Sec. 1,
        1995, pp 240.
[17]   Gilbert, J. L., and Buckley, C. A., "Mechanical-Electrochemical Interactions
        During In-vitro Fretting Corrosion Tests of Modular Taper Connections," Total
        Hip Revision Surgery, Raven Press, Ltd., New York, 1995, pp 41-50.
[18]   Yao, L. A., Gan, F. X., Zhao, Y. X., Yao, C. L., and Bear, J. L., "Microelectrode
        Monitoring the Crevice Corrosion of Titanium," Corrosion, Vol. 47, 1991, pp
        420-423.

[19]   Rostoker, W., Pretzel, C. W., and Galante, J. O., "Couple Corrosion Among Alloys for Skeletal Prostheses," Journal of Biomedical Materials Research, Vol. 8, 1974, pp 407-419.

[20]   Rostoker, W., Galante, J. O., and Lereim, P., "Evaluation of Couple/Crevice Corrosion by Prosthetic Alloys Under In-vivo Conditions," Journal of Biomedical Materials Research, Vol. 12, 1978, pp 823-829.

[21]   Kummer, F. J., and Rose, R. M., "Corrosion of Titanium/Cobalt Chromium Alloy Couples," Journal of Bone and Joint Surgery, Vol. 8, 1983, pp 1125-1126.

[22]   Kawalec, J. S., Brown, S. A., Payer, J. H., and Merritt, K., "Mixed Metal Fretting Corrosion of Ti-6Al-4V and Wrought Cobalt Alloy," Journal of Biomedical Materials Research, Vol. 29, 1995, pp 867-873.

[23]   Gilbert, J. L., Buckley, C. A., and Lautenschlager, E. P., "Titanium Oxide Film Fracture and Repassivation: The Effect of Potential, pH, and Aeration," Medical Applications of Titanium and Its Alloys: The Materials and Biological Issues, ASTM STP 1272, S. A. Brown and J. E. Lemons, Eds., American Society for Testing and Materials, Philadelphia, PA, 1996.

[24]   Goldberg, J. R., Gilbert, J. L., and Lautenschlager, E. P., "Electrochemical Behavior of CoCrMo Alloy After Mechanical Fracture of the Surface Oxide Film," Transactions of the Society for Biomaterials, Society for Biomaterials, Minneapolis, MN, Vol. 18, 1995, pg. 206.

Richard D. Lambert[1] and Terry W. McLean[2]

TEST METHOD COMPARING TORSIONAL FATIGUE OF MODULAR ACETABULAR COMPONENTS

REFERENCE: Lambert, R.D., and McLean, T.W., "**Test Method Comparing Torsional Fatigue of Modular Acetabular Components,**" *Modularity of Orthopedic Implants, ASTM STP 1301,* Donald E. Marlowe, Jack E. Parr, and Michael B. Mayor, Eds., American Society for Testing and Materials, 1997.

Abstract: The acetabular component is the focus of new testing methods dedicated to the development of improved total hip prostheses. Test methods had previously been developed to assess the performance of the femoral component in both the static and dynamic modes. These methods were designed in accordance with standards generated by such organizations as ASTM, ISO, and by research institutions. However, acetabular components were generally tested in the static mode to evaluate engagement strength and torsional resistance of the liner. While these tests are important and give a measure of the mechanical integrity of the device, they do not fully address clinical performance.

From retrieved components, it appears that a loose or failing locking mechanism allows torsional forces to transfer through the liner causing liner abrasion, burnishing, and in some cases degradation of the locking mechanism itself. Success of the device may be further compromised by the biological response to debris created by micromotion between the mating components. This study was undertaken to assess the rotational stability of the acetabular liner in a dynamic mode. Several acetabular component designs were torsionally fatigued at ±2.5 Nm at a rate of 3-5 hertz for 10 million cycles. The test components exhibited liner micromotion ranging from 0.059° to 2.89°, and damage to the nonarticulating interface and locking mechanism of tested liners was visually identified.

This method for dynamic testing of acetabular components provides an understanding of the performance of the device under torsional fatigue conditions. It demonstrates the importance of a rotationally stable liner, as damage to the nonarticulating interface of tested liners is similar to damage reported in the literature for retrieved components. Further, it determines the endurance of the liner locking mechanism when subjected to dynamic torsional forces.

KEYWORDS: total hip arthroplasty, acetabular, micromotion, wear, polyethylene

---

[1] Senior Research Engineer, Orthopaedic Research, Smith & Nephew Orthopaedics, 1450 Brooks Road, Memphis, Tennessee 38116
[2] Senior Research Technician, Orthopaedic Research, Smith & Nephew Orthopaedics, 1450 Brooks Road, Memphis, Tennessee 38116

BACKGROUND

Total hip arthroplasty involves reconstruction of the proximal femur and acetabulum to treat painful arthritis, traumatic injury, and other degenerative joint diseases [1]. The first modular acetabular prosthesis, consisting of a metal shell and a polyethylene insert, was introduced by Harris in 1970 [2]. Since that time, modular acetabular components have offered the flexibility to custom-fit prostheses intraoperatively, saving time and expense. They have also allowed physicians the option of revising only part of the acetabular component in the event of revision surgery.

However, modular pieces must be carefully designed and manufactured to prevent fretting or disassociation. In fact, one of the most critical issues confronting the orthopaedic community is the body's reaction to wear debris generated at the metal/polyethylene interface of acetabular components. Although polyethylene particles are assumed to be generated at the articulating interface of the femoral ball and polyethylene liner, studies have shown that articulation between the liner and shell may occur with some designs [3,4,5,6,7,8]. Problems associated with articulation between the liner and shell include fretting or burnishing of the liner dome and failure of the locking mechanism.

A review of the literature indicates that most test methods for acetabular components were developed to measure load to failure in a static mode, producing disassociation or mechanical failure of the device. However, these tests do not replicate the kind of clinical damage which has been reported. From retrieved components, it appears that torsional forces transferred to the liner cause liner micromotion, abrasion, burnishing, and in some cases degradation of the locking mechanism itself.

OBJECTIVE

This test method was developed to quantify the rotational displacement between the liner and shell under simulated in vivo torque loading, evaluate the integrity of the liner locking mechanism, and to identify cumulative damage occurring at the liner/shell interface.

METHOD

Acetabular Component Preparation

Six acetabular components ranging from 52 - 60 mm and designed by different manufacturers were obtained for this evaluation. All components were new and considered to be of implant quality.

The liners of the test components were carefully prepared for testing by drilling a 1.70 mm diameter hole into the rim of the liner at the midpoint of the wall for placement of a linear variable displacement transducer (LVDT) reference marker. The liners were then coated with a thin layer of gold on the nonarticulating surface (>5 microns) using a Desk II Sputter Coater (Denton Vaccum, Inc., Cherryhill, NJ), to enhance the visualization of abrasive wear on the liner surface after testing.

The acetabular shells were fixed in a metal potting fixture with bone cement (Palacos R®, Smith & Nephew Richards Inc.). Fixation holes on the shells were sealed using bakers clay, so that cement would not be allowed to interfere with the inner diameter surface of the shell. The shells were then mounted on a Bionix 810 (MTS Corporation, Minneapolis, MN) test frame in a fixture which was designed to hold the face of the shell perpendicular to the axis of rotation, and lowered into the bone cement to at least two-thirds of their radius until the bone cement cured.

After the bone cement had cured, the liners were locked into the shells following as closely as possible the manufacturers' specifications. Once the liner was inserted, a 1.78 mm diameter pin was press-fit into its predrilled hole. The pin acted as a referencing post for an LVDT.

Assembly/Mounting of Test Construct

A femoral head was used to transfer the torque and load directly to the liner and the liner locking mechanism. The head was glass-beaded and a series of small-diameter divots was randomly drilled into the articulating surface of the liner to improve the adhesiveness between the liner and head. The liner was not penetrated while drilling. Plastic steel putty (Devcon, Danvers, MA) was applied to the articulating surface of the liner. The head was attached to a neck taper and placed in the upper ram of the Bionix test frame. The head was lowered into the liner and loaded to 89 N until the plastic steel putty cured.

The acetabular construct was then mounted to the Bionix. An LVDT, model LBB-375-TA-100, (Schaevitz, Pennsauken, NJ) was secured to the test frame and placed perpendicular to the 1.78 mm (0.070 in.) diameter pin to measure displacement of the liner relative to the metal shell. A Microprocessor 2000 (Schaevitz, Pennsauken, NJ) provided the necessary voltage to drive the LVDT, and an HP Plotter 7090A (Hewlett Packard, San Diego, CA) recorded LVDT output over 12 to 24-hour intervals. A schematic of the mounted acetabular component and test set-up is given in Figure 1.

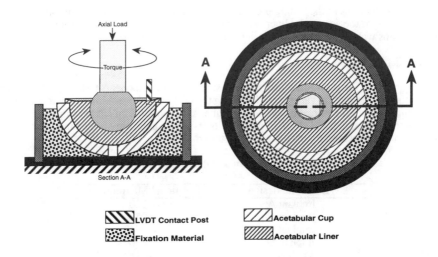

FIG. 1--Schematic of the mounted acetabular construct

Cyclic Loading

During the walk cycle, frictional torque is generated by the articulation of the head against the acetabular component. Davidson et al. reported the frictional torque for a 28 mm Co-Cr femoral head to be 2.5 Nm [9]. Using 2.5 Nm as the maximum torque, a cyclic sinusoidal torsional load (±2.5 Nm) was applied to the acetabular component at a rate ranging from 3 to 5 hertz, depending on the displacement of the liner. Concurrent with the torsional load, an axial compression load of 222.4 N was applied to the acetabular component. The static load provided axial stability for the liner for the duration of the study. The liner was fatigued for 10 million cycles or until progressive micromotion ceased.

Liner Disassembly

Liners were disassembled according to manufacturers' specifications whenever possible. In some cases, the design of the axial locking mechanism would not allow for conventional disengagement because of damage that may have resulted in distracting the liner from the shell. These components often utilized a locking ring for axial stability. For disassembly, the ring was located on the outer surface of the shell prior to testing, and was machined away at the conclusion of the test. This task was accomplished by placing the cylinder of bone cement in a lathe and carefully cutting the ring from the shell. In this manner, the nonarticulating interface was not damaged as a result of disassembly.

Micromotion Normalization

To normalize the micromotion measured for the various acetabular components, linear displacements taken from the LVDT were used to calculate corresponding angular displacements. By comparing angular displacements, the various acetabular designs could be evaluated relative to micromotion.

RESULTS

The three objectives of the testing protocol were accomplished during this investigation. Micromotion of the acetabular liner was measured, the integrity of the various locking mechanisms was evaluated, and abrasion/damage of the liner surface was observed.

Liner Micromotion

Micromotion of the acetabular liner was measured for all components tested; however, the magnitude of the motion varied greatly among the designs. The maximum micromotion determined for all the implants was 2.89° of liner excursion in Implant D. Implant B exhibited the least amount of micromotion with 0.059°. Table 1 gives the maximum micromotion measured for each component tested.

TABLE 1--Maximum acetabular liner micromotion

Acetabular design	Rotational Micromotion
Implant A	1.120°
Implant B	0.059°
Implant C	0.354°
Implant D	2.890°
Implant E	0.718°
Implant F	1.300°

In Figure 2, acetabular liner micromotion is shown relative to elapsed time. Most liners tested were subjected to fatigue for 10 million cycles. Those that were fatigued for fewer than 10 million cycles either had a locking mechanism failure or the test was stopped due to nonprogressive micromotion.

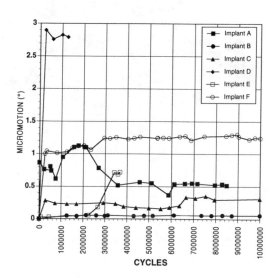

FIG. 2--Micromotion vs. time

Liner Locking Mechanism

The rotational locking mechanism of Implant D failed after 1.1 million cycles. Figure 3 shows the metal pin which provided the rotational stability for the liner had dislodged from the liner and displaced between the liner and shell. This implant was the only one showing structural failure of the rotational locking mechanism.

Liner Wear

Abrasion or wear was observed on the nonarticulating interface of all of the acetabular liners tested. Most of the wear occurred on the dome of the liner or around the liner rim, as shown in Figures 4 and 5, respectively. One acetabular component exhibited significant wear at the locking mechanism. (Fig. 6)

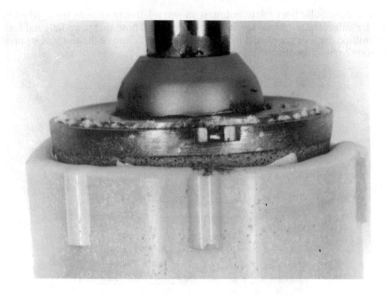

FIG. 3--Implant D with failed rotational stabilizing pin

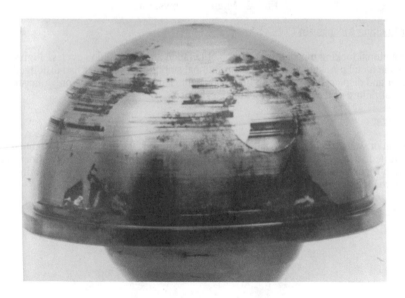

FIG. 4--Implant E with wear on the dome

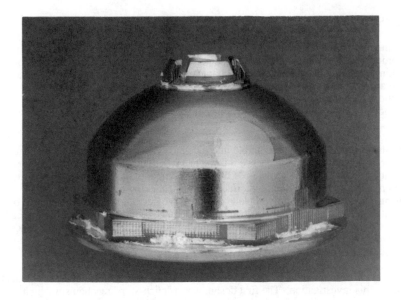

FIG. 5--Implant A with wear on the rim

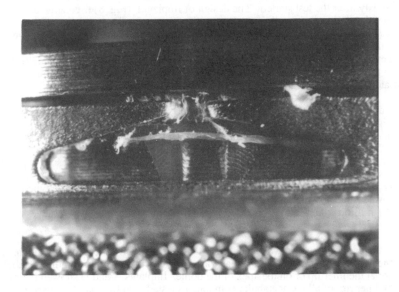

FIG. 6--Implant E with wear at the locking mechanism

DISCUSSION

This test method simulates in vivo torsional loading conditions placed on the acetabular liner in order to measure liner micromotion, determine the effect of torsional loading on the liner locking mechanism, and assess wear characteristics of the nonarticulating interface. All of the acetabular designs evaluated in this investigation exhibited some degree of micromotion; therefore, it is important to evaluate the effects of micromotion on the performance of the implant, as well as to consider the clinical effects of the resulting wear debris.

In acetabular components, the articulating interface has often been perceived to be the only contributor of polyethylene debris, since it is the site where the femoral and acetabular components meet and force is transferred from one component to the other. However, wear patterns on the nonarticulating interface and loose locking mechanisms on retrieved components have proved that polyethylene debris is also generated at other interfaces of the component. Collier and Bobyn have documented damage to the back side of the liner as the result of articulation between the acetabular liner and shell. The clinical significance of this damage is the possible premature failure of the locking mechanism, as well as the wear debris generated and its association with an immune system response.

Two types of rotational locking mechanisms were identified for the acetabular components evaluated in this investigation. The first design was a "click-stop" mechanism which achieved rotational stability from the interference of two similar geometries, such as the scallop design of Implant C (Fig. 7) or a hexagon like Implant A (Fig. 5). The components that had a "click-stop" lock mechanism seemed to allow for various degrees of micromotion by design, probably to ensure that they assembled easily and that axial locking strength was not compromised. Micromotion was measured for the "click-stop" components almost instantaneously after the test started. The design of Implant F (Fig. 8) used a metal post on the shell rim that fit between scalloped edges on the liner to provide rotatory stability. Implant D (Fig. 3) achieved rotational stability by using a metal peg pressed into the liner that protruded through a slot in the shell. This particular component is the only design that failed structurally during the test. After 1.1 million cycles, the metal peg dislodged from its position in the liner and jammed in between the liner and the shell wall. This implant also demonstrated the greatest degree of micromotion of the implants tested (2.89°).

The second type of locking mechanism used barbs or tynes to secure the liner rotationally. These designs rely on sharp points that grab and deform the polyethylene liner. The barbed lock mechanism produced the least micromotion of the components evaluated in this study, with 0.059° measured. The design of Implant B (Fig. 9) used four barbs that cut a groove in the liner as it was assembled to provide rotational stability. The tyned design depends on five sets of pointed tynes, like the ones shown in Figures 4 and 6, to grip the liner by deforming the polyethylene around the tyne. Unlike other designs studied, the tyned design showed relatively no micromotion initially. However, significant micromotion did occur at 2.1 million cycles, and progressed through 3.5 million cycles, when the test was stopped.

All the acetabular components evaluated during this investigation exhibited some degree of wear on the nonarticulating interface. Wear was specific to two locations on the acetabular liner; either at the liner lip or on the apex of the dome. Implants A and D showed the most wear at the liner rim of all the acetabular components tested. On Implant A, a discernible groove was observed on the rim which was caused by the cyclic rotation of the liner inside the shell. The groove actually decreased liner micromotion over time as sufficient material was removed to create a new locking groove. Implants D,E, and F displayed the most abrasive wear on the liner dome during this study, and are shown in Figures 10,4, and 8, respectively.

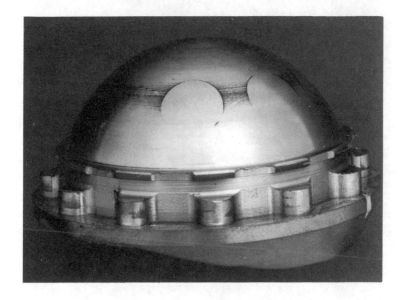

FIG. 7--Implant C after fatigue testing

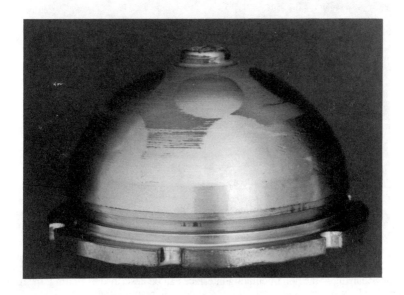

FIG. 8--Implant F after fatigue testing

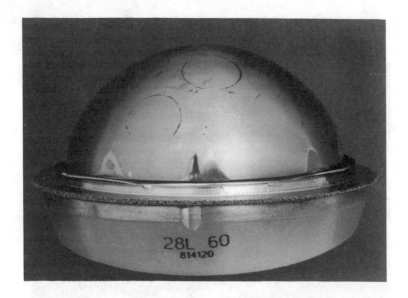

FIG. 9--Implant B after fatigue testing

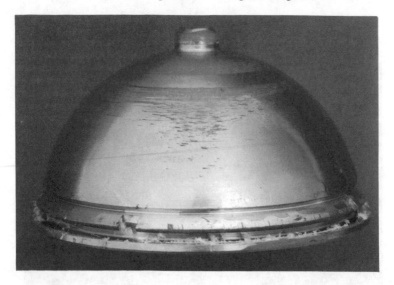

FIG. 10--Implant D after fatigue testing

The wear occurring at the nonarticulating interface can be described as fretting, the relative micromotion between two opposing surfaces which can result in the mechanical degradation of one or both surfaces. Generally, the amount of fretting can be correlated to the magnitude of micromotion occurring between the two surfaces; the greater the micromotion the greater the wear debris produced, and the lesser the micromotion the lesser the wear debris produced. The results obtained in this evaluation follow the same principle. Acetabular components with greater degrees of micromotion displayed more surface damage than those with less micromotion. Designs that reduce the production of wear debris by providing a stable acetabular liner, axially and rotationally, increase the longevity of the implant. Loose liners, failed liner locking mechanisms, and wear tracks on the back side of the liner, similar to what has been observed here, have been presented clinically through retrieved acetabular components.

This torsional fatigue evaluation uses information gained from retrieved components to produce a test method which measures the rotational stability of the liner locking mechanism, and qualitatively assesses the wear characteristics of the nonarticulating interface.

CONCLUSIONS

This fatigue test for the modular acetabular component attempts to re-create the in vivo torsional loading conditions placed on the liner in order to measure the liner micromotion and qualitatively determine the degree of wear on the nonarticulating interface. The wear patterns on the nonarticulating interfaces obtained in this investigation are similar to those documented in the literature, indicating that rotational micromotion has a key role in the wear debris generated from the back side of the liner. Furthermore, this method provides an avenue for evaluating the mechanical integrity of an acetabular component's rotational locking mechanism under high cycle fatigue.

REFERENCES

[1]   Harkess J.W., "Arthroplasty of the Hip," Campbell's Operative Orthopaedics, Vol. 1, 1992.

[2]   Harris, W.H., "A New Total Hip Implant," Clinical Orthopaedics and Related Research, No. 81, November-December 1971, pp. 105-113.

[3]   Bobyn, J.D., Collier, J.P., Mayor, M.B., McTighe, T., Tanzer, M., Vaughn, B.K., "Particulate Debris in Total Hip Arthroplasty: Problems and Solutions," Scientific Exhibit at the 1993 AAOS Meeting, San Francisco, CA.

[4]   Collier, J.P., Mayor, M.B., Jensen, R.E., Surprenant, V.A., Suprenant, H.P., McNamara, J.L., and Belec, L.B., "Mechanisms of Failure of Modular Prostheses," Clinical Orthopaedics and Related Research, Number 285, December 1992, pp. 129-139.

[5]   Huk, O.L., Bansal, M., Betts, F., Lieberman, J.R., Huo, M.H., and Salvati, E.A., "Generation of Polyethylene and Metal Debris from Cementless Modular Acetabular Components in Total Hip Arthroplasty," 39th Annual Meeting, Orthopaedic Research Society, February 15-18, 1993, San Francisco, CA.

[6]   Huk, O.L., Bansal, M., Betts, F., Rimnac, C.M., Lieberman, J.R., Huo, M.H., and Salvati, E.A., "Polyethylene and Metal Debris Generated by Non-Articulating Surfaces of Modular Acetabular Components," The Journal of Bone and Joint Surgery, Vol. 76-B, No. 4, July 1994, pp. 568-574.

[7]   Maloney, W.J. and Jasti, M., " Wear Debris in Total Hip Arthroplasty," Seminars in Arthroplasty, Vol. 4, No. 3, July 1993, pp 125-135.

[8]   Maloney, W.J., Peters, P., Engh, C.A., and Chandler, H., "Severe Osteolysis of the Pelvis in Association with Acetabular Replacement without Cement," The Journal of Bone and Joint Surgery, Vol. 75-A, No. 11, November 1993, pp. 1627-1635.

[9]   Davidson, J.A. and Brasher, T. "The Effect of Femoral Head Size and Material on the Frictional Moment During Torque," Proceedings from the 1989 A.S.M.E Winter Symposium- The Mechanics of Joints, December 10-15, 1989.

Stanley A. Brown[1], Alula Abera[2], Mark D'Onofrio[3], and Curt Flemming[3]

EFFECTS OF NECK EXTENSION, COVERAGE, AND FREQUENCY ON THE FRETTING
CORROSION OF MODULAR THR BORE AND CONE INTERFACE

REFERENCE: Brown, S. A., Abera, A., D'Onofrio, M., and Flemming, C.,
"**Effects of Neck Extension, Coverage, and Frequency on the Fretting Corrosion
of Modular THR Bore and Cone Interface,**" *Modularity of Orthopedic Implants,
ASTM STP 1301,* Donald E. Marlowe, Jack E. Parr, and Michael B. Mayor, Eds.,
American Society for Testing and Materials, 1997.

ABSTRACT: Examination of retrieved modular total hip replacements
(THR's) has identified fretting corrosion as one of the principal
mechanisms of implant corrosion at the bore and cone interface.
Increased instability due to increased neck extension has been
attributed to one of the design factors affecting corrosion rates. A
series of experiments was conducted on THR's with cobalt chromium
molybdenum alloy heads and Ti 6Al 4V stems, which demonstrated higher
fretting corrosion currents with longer neck extensions. Shortening the
skirt reduced corrosion rates. In a second series, the effects of wave
form and cycling frequency demonstrated higher currents with a ramp
versus a sine wave, and higher currents with higher frequencies.
Examination of the frequency components of the Paul curve for loads on
the hip during gait demonstrated that higher frequencies may be
appropriate for device testing.

KEY WORDS: fretting corrosion, Ti 6Al 4V, CoCrMo alloy, mixed metal,
Modular total hips, frequency

The development of modular total hip replacements (THR's)
permitted the use of heads and stems of different materials, so as to
optimize the properties of each component. One of the clinical
advantages of modular total hips is the option to use heads with
different lengths of neck extension, so as to better fit the prosthesis
to the patient without expense of maintaining large implant inventories.
However, the advent of modularity was not without reports of clinical
complications attributed to interfacial corrosion [1,2]. Early reports
on analysis of retrieved implants identified corrosion to be limited to

[1] Biomedical engineer, FDA/CDRH/DMMS, 12200 Wilkins Ave.,
Rockville, MD 20852.

[2] COSTEP, FDA/CDRH/DMMS, present address: student, Department of
Mechanical Engineering, MIT, Cambridge MA 02139

[3]Student, Department of Biomedical Engineering, Case Western
Reserve University, Cleveland OH 44106.

devices with dissimilar metals [3,4]. Subsequent retrieval studies have suggested fretting as an initiator of corrosion of modular hips [5,6,7,8]. Corrosion was been seen with both mixed and similar metal devices. Examination of the correlation between bore and cone corrosion and neck extension of retrieved prostheses suggested more corrosion with the longer necks [5,6,9]. Part of the concern is that the corrosion products in the form of chromium orthophosphates may contribute to local tissue reactions, as well as exacerbate the problem of polymeric wear and osteolysis [10].

To study the effect of fretting in modular THR corrosion in the laboratory, a test method was developed [11,12,13] to measure currents associated with cyclically loading an inverted prosthesis in a saline bath. Preliminary studies *in vitro* demonstrated a similar correlation between corrosion and neck extension, as was seen with retrieved specimens. These results led to the more detailed studies on the effects of neck extension and coverage presented in the present report.

A screw drive universal testing machine was utilized in these studies. This device applied a cyclic load in the form of a ramp; i.e. fixed cross head speed in both the up and down direction. More recent studies have been conducted using a servohydraulic system, with which the loading pattern and frequency can be controlled. Differences observed in current recordings suggested an investigation to compare ramp and sine wave loading patterns.

In consideration of test protocols for testing modular devices, one also needs to consider the normal activities of daily living (ADL's). A person does not walk continuously for 10 million cycles. In fact, ADL's are a series of short events. Walking to the bath room or getting a cup of coffee probably takes fewer than 50 cycles; walking around our laboratory building takes 230 cycles. Walking a mile takes about 1000 cycles. To this end, the present studies also examined the fretting corrosion of modular THR's in a series of short "walks".

The use of a servohydraulic system also presents the opportunity to address the question of what is the most appropriate frequency for simulating gait. The classic studies by Paul [14,15] demonstrated a rather complicated, bimodal loading pattern on the hip joint. While the gait is simulated as one cycle per second, the wave form pattern actually contains several higher frequency components. To this end, the Paul curve has been examined for frequency.

The objectives of present studies were to investigate the effects of different neck extension and skirt configurations on the fretting corrosion of the bore and cone interface of modular hips. The effects of loading wave form, number of cycles, and frequency were also examined.

METHODS

Implants donated by several manufacturers were mounted in an inverted position as described previously [11]. The heads were placed on the stems and firmly set in place by hand, without impaction with a mallet. They were then placed in a 0.9% saline bath with the fluid level 2-3 mm above the bore and cone interface. To insure that the measurements were solely that of interface fretting, the head and its articulation was insulated with a rubber skirt, or a section of bicycle inner tube. A zero resistance ammeter (Keithley 486) was used to measure fretting corrosion currents between the prosthesis and a commercial pure titanium counter electrode with a surface area comparable to that of the femoral stem. Currents were recorded with a strip chart recorder (Linear) and a digital storage oscilloscope (Tektronix 7704).

Studies of neck extension and coverage were conducted with a screw drive universal testing machine (Scott GRE 1000). Implants were loaded at a rate of 0.5 cycles per second, at a load of 0-2000 N. Tests were run for 12 minutes (360 cycles) and the last five current cycles averaged for a data point. Each study consisted of 5 tests, from which the mean and standard deviation were calculated. Studies on wave form and frequency were conducted on a servohydraulic test machine (MTS 458) at a load of 40-1780 N. Several types of experimental protocols were used, as is described subsequently.

Neck Extension

As is shown in Figures 1 and 2, the terms "extension", "penetration", and "coverage" were used to describe relationship between the head position on the cone. In designing a modular hip system, the manufacturers define a head position relative to the stem as a "0 mm" neck extension. From that they modify the head geometry such that the center of the head is either further from, or closer to the stem. Heads are available with positive and negative extensions, expressed in millimeters. To compare the relationship between the head and stem of different modular designs in terms of how far the cone penetrates the spherical portion of the head, we used the term "penetration" to describe the location of the cone end relative to the center of the ball, expressed in units of the head radius. A penetration of "1.0 R" would mean that the cone penetrated 1 radius into the head, i.e. it penetrated to the center of the ball. Cones with penetrations greater that 1.0 R went deeper than the center; cones with penetrations of less than 1.0 R did not penetrate to the center. "Coverage" was expressed in millimeters as the length of cone covered by the head and the neck extension or skirt.

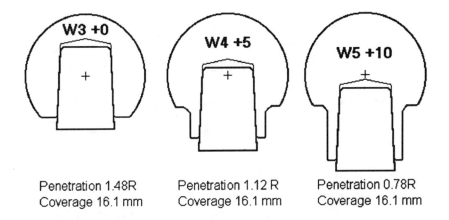

Penetration 1.48R   Penetration 1.12 R   Penetration 0.78R
Coverage 16.1 mm   Coverage 16.1 mm   Coverage 16.1 mm

Figure 1. Penetration and Coverage for "W" THR's with neck extensions of +0, +5mm and +10mm.

Studies were conducted with identical hips in each series, but with neck extensions; when available extensions of +0mm, +5mm, and +10mm were used. The nomenclature used in these studies, as shown in Figures 1 and 2 is a letter-number code. The letter identifies the manufacturer. The letters do not represent the first letter of the manufacturer, so as to maintain their anonymity and avoid comparisons

between products. Anonymity is essential since some of the devices
tested were specially prepared for studies addressing a specific
question, and may not represent standard commercially available
products. The first number was assigned sequentially to the stem tested
from that manufacturer; "W3" was the third stem tested from manufacturer
"W". The second number was the head extension.

Three series of modular hips were studied for the effects of neck
extension: 2 device designs from "W" and one from "S". The design
parameters fare summarized in Table 1. As is shown in Figure 1,
increasing the neck extension of the "W" implant design did not change
the amount of coverage, or contact area between bore and cone, but it
did result in decreasing the amount of the cone that was within the
spherical part of the head. The "S" series coverage also remained
constant at 14.5 mm. The penetrations for the +0, +5 and +10 heads were
1.38R, 1.02R and 0.66R, respectively.

Cone Coverage

To study the effects of coverage, two +10 mm extension heads were
modified by cutting off part of the skirt, such that the surface area of
the cone covered by the sleeve was reduced by 25% and 50% of that of the
unmodified head. This did not change the relationship between the
spherical portion of the ball and the cone, as shown in Figure 2.

Cone Penetration

The cone of one hip was cut to reduce the amount of coverage, and
the amount that the cone penetrated into the head. As shown in Figure
2, the cone was cut such that it was outside of the spherical portion of
the head, with a penetration of 0.33 R and a coverage of 40% less than
control.

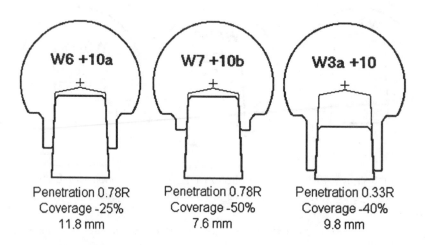

Figure 2. Reduction of cone coverage of −25% and −50% by cutting the
skirts, and reduction of penetration by cutting the cone.

TABLE 1. Summary of the design parameters for the heads studied. Data
are expressed as "coverage / penetration"

Test Head Diameter	"W" 1st series 32 mm	"W" 2nd series 28 mm	"S" series 32 mm
+0 mm	14.6/1.40R	16.1/1.48R	14.5/1.38R
+5 mm		16.1/1.12R	14.5/1.02R
+10 mm	14.9/0.80R	16.1/0.78R	14.5/0.66R
+10 mm, -25% coverage		11.8/0.78R	
+10 mm, -50% coverage		7.6/0.78R	
+10 mm, Reduced penetration		9.8/0.33R	

RESULTS

Effects of Neck Extension and Cone Coverage

The results for all three series of studies demonstrated
significantly higher fretting corrosion currents with increasing neck
extension, as shown in Table 2. Reducing the coverage significantly
reduced the fretting corrosion currents as shown in the table.

TABLE 2. Fretting corrosion currents (μA) expressed as mean ± standard
deviation.

Test Neck Extension	"W" 1st series	"W" 2nd series	"S" series
+0 mm	0.5 ± 0.1	1.7 ± 0.4	0.6 ± 0.2
+5 mm		3.9 ± 0.4	1.0 ± 0.2
+10 mm	9.1 ± 1.2	8.3 ± 0.1	9.4 ± 1.4
+10 mm, -25% coverage		7.2 ± 0.7	
+10 mm, -50% coverage		1.6 ± 0.1	
+10 mm, Reduced penetration		4.3 ± 2.2	

Effects of Cone Penetration

This modification of reduced penetration resulted in an initially
very unstable interface. At the beginning of each test, the currents
reached spikes as high as 75 μA compared to 8 μA for the unmodified
device. However, after a period of several minutes, the currents
dropped to a level comparable to that of the +5 mm neck extension.

Effects of Wave Form

Short term studies were conducted to compare fretting corrosion
currents of a hip loaded with a ramp at 1 Hz for 100 cycles, followed by
a short pause and then 100 cycles with a sine wave loading pattern. In a

given session, this pattern was repeated several times, simulating a series of short 2 minute 40 second walks. As can be seen in Figure 3, the current increased more rapidly, and to a higher level with the ramp as compared to the sine. During the pause, the current rapidly dropped, indicating repassivation of the interface surfaces.

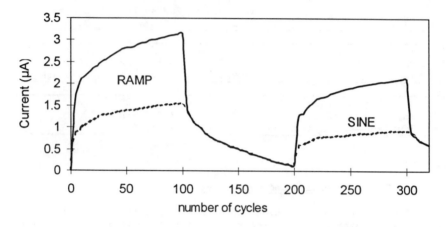

Figure 3. Corrosion currents for ramp and sine wave loading at 1 cycle per second or 1 Hz. The solid (upper) line represents the maximum or peak currents for each cycle; the broken (lower) line represents the minimum current for each cycle.

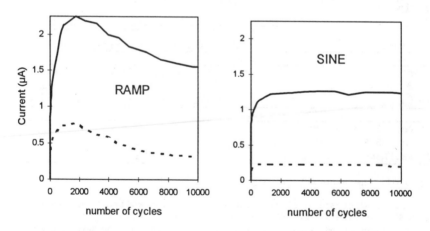

Figure 4. Peak to peak current envelopes for fretting corrosion currents versus number of cycles, for ramp and sine wave loading at 1 cycle per second, or 1 Hz.

After each pause, be it for several minutes, hours or days, the application of load always resulted in a rapid increase in current which reached a plateau. The studies done with the screw drive machine, and those with the servohydraulic ramp function typically showed an initial

increase, followed by a decrease to a stable plateau level, as shown in
Figure 4.   The 12 minute experimental protocol utilized with the screw
drive machine was based on the observation that the recordings had
reached a stable plateau by this time.

Effects of Frequency

A series of experiments was conducted to examine the effects of
frequency of a sine wave on the fretting corrosion currents. There was a
progressive increase in the current as frequency increased from 0.5 to
2.5 Hz, as shown in Figure 5.   A similar increase in current with
increasing frequency was also observed with analysis of these data at
100, 300, and 600 cycles.   A second series at these five frequencies was
run out to 2500 cycles.   The results also demonstrated a similar
frequency dependence.

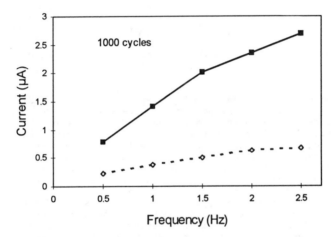

Figure 5.   Maximum and minimum (peak to peak) current values for
experiments conducted at 0.5, 1.0, 1.5, 2.0 and 2.5 Hz for 1000 cycles.

A third series conducted at frequencies of 2, 5, and 10 Hz showed
a similar increase in current with increasing frequency.   For
comparison, the 1000 cycle data are shown in Figure 6. While these data
can not be compared directly, since they represent different time
periods in the testing history of this device, they do show the same
trend.   These experiments were run out to 10,000 cycles with the same
results: current increases with increasing frequency.

DISCUSSION

These studies have demonstrated that modifications in the bore and
cone configuration, i.e. neck extension or coverage, have a significant
effect on fretting corrosion of the interface.   Increasing neck
extension resulted in higher fretting currents.   This could be due to
decreased cone penetration and increased bending moment.   Examination of
retrieved prostheses [5,9] revealed localization of damage patterns on
the bores and cones suggestive of bending of the cone due to the applied

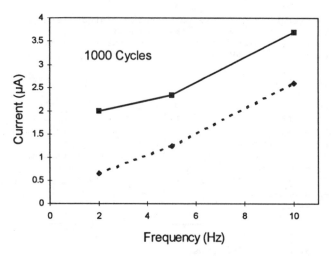

Figure 6. Maximum and minimum current values for fretting corrosion at
1000 cycles at 2 Hz, 5 Hz and 10 Hz.

forces during gait. Examination of current recordings [9,12] showed a
biphasic wave pattern also suggestive of cone bending. Current
increased suddenly toward the end of the loading phase of the cycle,
suggesting slipping of the interface. A second pulse was seen during
unloading, suggesting slipping of the interface as the cone straightened
out, or the head slipped back to its unloaded position.
     Decreasing coverage which did not change cone penetration did not
result in a change in critical load. However, the decrease in interface
surface area and the lack of the long sleeve did produce a decrease in
fretting current. It can be hypothesized that this was due to a shorter
length of coverage in which relative motion could occur. One of the most
clear demonstrations of the role of interface mechanics on fretting
corrosion was seen in the change of current wave forms with reduction of
the percent coverage. With full coverage the currents were high and the
wave form clearly biphasic. As the coverage was reduced, the currents
dropped, and the curves lost the biphasic nature. These indicate major
changes in interface dynamics. While these data suggest that short
skirts are better, they do not consider the strength of the interface in
terms of the force required to pull off the heads. The results seen
with shortening the cone support the hypothesis that cone penetration is
a critical issue.
     The differences seen between the ramp and sine data indicate a
significant role for frequency. The ramp loading rate is higher than
the sine for most of the cycle, and it has an abrupt transition between
loading and unloading. The frequency studies further demonstrate that
currents increase with increasing frequency. The short term 100 cycle
walk studies, and all other experiments demonstrate that the interface
rapidly repassivates at the end of a loading sequence. With initiation
of loading, currents rapidly increase. Since life is a series of short
walks, such short term studies may provide more insight into the
stability and dynamics of the modular interface, than would long term
studies.

A person may walk at one cycle per second, however, this does not imply that the forces about the hip joint can be represented by a 1 Hz sine wave. In his classic studies, Paul [14,15] used a force plate and gait analysis methods to calculate the force on the hip and other joints. The Paul curve as published in Dawson and Wright [15] was photo enlarged and digitized, as shown in Figure 7. A sine wave was added to the plot, with a program permitting adjustment of frequency and time shift. The first major increase in the Paul curve load, at about 0.1 second, represents heal strike. The large drop after the second large peak, at 0.6 seconds, is toe off. As seen in Figure 7, both these components closely match the 10 Hz sine wave. The periodicity, or frequency of the two major peaks themselves, are best approximated by a 2.4 Hz sine wave.

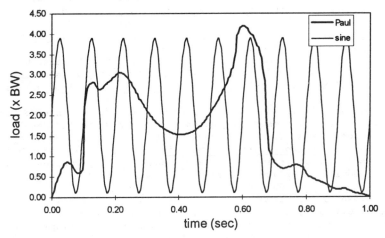

Figure 7. Load expressed as times body weight versus time for the Paul curve [9], and a superimposed 10 Hz sine wave. Note portions of the Paul curve that have similar slopes to the sine.

The Paul curve is based on normal walking speed of one cycle per second. However, it is not simulated with a 1 Hz sine wave. The frequency analysis data demonstrate that currents increase with increasing frequency. From these analyses, one may conclude that the use of frequencies higher that 1 Hz would be appropriate for testing modular devices. Studies with a Paul curve driving function are clearly indicated. Given that the same prostheses was used for all the wave form and frequency studies, and each experiment demonstrated the same transient response, even after many 100's of thousands of cycles, one might conclude that short term studies provide significant information regarding the stability of a modular interface and its susceptibility to fretting corrosion. However, it is not yet known how the magnitude of these fretting corrosion currents correlates with actual damage to the interface, and its clinical significance. For this, long term studies are indicated.

REFERENCES

1.   Svensson, O., Mathiesen, E.B., Reinholt, F.P., and Blomgren, G., "Formation of a Fulminant Soft-Tissue Pseudotumor after Uncemented Hip Arthroplasty", Journal of Bone and Joint Surgery, 70A: 1238-1242, 1988.
2.   Mathiesen, E.B., Lindgren, J.U., Blomgren, G.G.A., and Reinholt, F.P., "Corrosion of Modular Hip Prostheses", Journal of Bone and Joint Surgery, 73B: 569-575, 1991.
3.   Collier, J.P., Suprenant, V.A., Jensen, R.E., and Mayor, M.B., Corrosion at the Interface of Cobalt-alloy Heads on Titanium Alloy Stems", Clinical Orthopaedics 271: 305-312, 1991.
4.   Collier, J.P., Suprenant, V.A., Jensen, R.E., Mayor, M.B., and Suprenant, H.P., "Corrosion Between the Components of Modular Femoral Hip Prostheses', Journal of Bone and Joint Surgery, 74B: 511-517, 1992.
5.   Bauer, T.W., Brown, S.A., Jiang, M., Panigutti, M.A., and Flemming, C.A.C., "Corrosion of Modular Hip Stems", Transactions Orthopaedic Research Society 17:354, 1992.
6.   Brown, S.A., Flemming, C.A.C., Kawalec, J.S., Vassaux, C.J., Payer, J.H., Kraay, M.J., and Merritt, K., "Fretting Accelerated Crevice Corrosion of Modular Hips", Transactions Society for Biomaterials 15: 59, 1992.
7.   Gilbert, J.L., Buckley, C.A., and Jacobs, J.J., "In vivo Corrosion of Modular Hip Prosthesis Components in Mixed and Similar Metal Combinations. The Effects of Crevice, Stress, Motion, and Alloy Coupling", Journal of Biomedical Materials Research 27: 1533-1544, 1993.
8.   Cook, S.D., Barrack, R.L., and Clemow, A.J.T., "Corrosion and Wear at the Modular Interface of Uncemented Femoral Stems", Journal of Bone and Joint Surgery, 76B: 68-72, 1994.
9.   Brown, S.A., Flemming, C.A.C., Kawalec, J.S., Placko, H.E., Vassaux, C., Merritt, K., Payer, J.H., and Kraay, M.J., Fretting Corrosion Accelerates Crevice Corrosion of Modular Hip Tapers. Journal of Applied Biomaterials. 6: 19-26, 1995.
10.   Urban, R., Jacobs, J.J., Gilbert, J.L., and Galante, J.O., "Migration of Corrosion Products from Modular Hip Prostheses. Particle Microanalysis and Histopathological Findings", Journal of Bone and Joint Surgery, 76A: 1345-1359, 1994.
11.   Flemming, C.A.C., Brown, S.A., and Payer, J.H., "The use of Fretting Currents to Examine the Issues of Tolerances in Modular Hips", Transactions Society for Biomaterials 16: 275, 1993.
12.   Flemming, C.A.C., Brown, S.A., and Payer, J.H., "Mechanical Testing for Fretting Corrosion of Modular Total Hip Tapers", Biomaterials' Mechanical Properties. ASTM STP 1173, H.E. Kambic and A.T. Yokobori, Jr., Eds, American Society for Testing and Materials, Philidelphis, 1994, pp. 156-166.
13.   Brown, S.A., Flemming, C.A.C., and Payer, J.H., "Modifications of Head Neck Extension and Taper Angle Mismatch to Reduce Fretting Corrosion of Modular Total Hips, Transactions Orthopaedic Research Society 19: 593, 1994.
14.   Paul J. P. "Forces Transmitted by Joints in the Human Body", Proc Inst of Mech Engineers 181 (3J) paper 8, 1966.
15.   Johnson, G.R., "The Application of Basic Mechanics to the Human Body", Introduction to Bio-mechanics of Joints and Joint replacement, D. Dawson and V. Wright, Eds, Mechanical Engineering Publications, Ltd. London, 1981, p. 28.

Dominic R. Fosco[1] and Dennis J. Buchanan[1]

The Importance of Fatigue Loading When Assessing Liner/Shell Distraction Resistance and Congruency for Modular Acetabular Components

REFERENCE: Fosco, D. R. and Buchanan, D. J., "**The Importance of Fatigue Loading When Assessing Liner/Shell Distraction Resistance and Congruency for Modular Acetabular Components,**" *Modularity of Orthopedic Implants, ASTM STP 1301,* Donald E. Marlowe, Jack E. Parr, and Michael B. Mayor, Eds., American Society for Testing and Materials, 1997.

ABSTRACT: Modular acetabular components are now widely used in total hip arthroplasty (THA). A primary performance requirement for these two-piece acetabular cup designs is to maintain *in vivo* locking integrity between the polyethylene liner and the metal acetabular shell. Standards have been proposed that include the measurement of static push-out and lever-out forces to evaluate the mechanical integrity between the shell and liner. However, there are many variables that may affect *in vivo* performance. A modification of the proposed test standards is recommended to include moderate fatigue cycling, since fatigue has a demonstrated effect on distraction resistance and the potential for *in vivo* disassembly.

KEYWORDS: implant, prosthesis, total hip arthroplasty, THA, acetabular cup, modular

A current trend in total hip arthroplasty includes the use of modular components to facilitate surgery and to minimize the requirement to have large inventories of different size components available in the surgical suite. Although modularity has positive benefits, a primary design consideration must be to maintain integrity of the assembled components *in vivo*. For this reason, it is essential to have testing standards that effectively evaluate various designs and that attempt to predict performance of the components in the clinical environment.

There are reports in the clinical literature of disassociation of two-piece acetabular cup systems and for biomechanical testing that supposedly predicts *in vivo* locking integrity between the plastic acetabular cup liner and the corresponding metal shell [1]. Standard test methods have also been drafted to bring consistency and uniformity to the evaluation of various designs, but these standards may fail to take into account all of the critical variables affecting disassembly in clinical use (Draft Standard Test Method for Static Evaluation of Liner Locking Mechanism—Push-out Test, ASTM Task Force F04.22.17, 1994 and Draft Standard Test Method for Determination of the Lever-out Strength of Acetabular Shell/Liner Assemblies, ASTM Task Force F04.22.17, 1994).

---

[1]Applied Technology Group, Research and Development, Wright Medical chnology, Inc., Arlington, TN 38002.

There are several variables that may affect performance of two-piece acetabular cup system locking integrity, including but not limited to:

- Design
- Fatigue
- Surgical technique
- Creep
- Sterilization
- Processing and the resulting properties of the ultra-high molecular weight polyethylene (UHMWPE).

This paper focuses on the effect of fatigue and proposes that moderate fatigue cycling be considered as an integral part of the standard test methods.

Objectives

This study was undertaken for the following reasons:

1. To present data to show that fatigue cycling (or moderate "break-in" of acetabular components) can affect performance test values for congruency, push-out, and lever-out.

2. To suggest that fatigue cycling be introduced as an integral part of the "Standard Test Methods" for these components to ensure that test evaluations of acetabular cup systems are sufficiently rigorous.

A moderate amount of fatigue cycling may change the "push-out" and "lever-out" test results that are now being reported in the literature for various two-piece acetabular cup designs. Our objective was to measure percent change in push-out and lever-out values after fatigue cycling. The results would confirm that fatigue cycling should be conducted before cup/liner integrity tests (push-out and lever-out) to get values that would be more representative of *in vivo* conditions. More importantly, adopting this method into standard test methods would help to ensure that design integrity is maintained after "break-in" or moderate fatigue cycling.

Clinical Relevance

The measured values for cup/liner integrity may give a false sense of design security (or design safety factor) if the evaluation is done without subjecting the assembly to fatigue cycling that would tend to seat or "break in" the components. Thus, if a design could potentially lose a significant percentage of its locking mechanism integrity, as measured during post-fatigue testing, it would not be acceptable for clinical application.

A value of 2,000 fatigue cycles represents about one day of normal walking (assuming 1,000,000 cycles per year) and is deemed sufficient to evaluate initial "break-in" of the components. Long-term fatigue is beyond the scope of this study.

Push-out and lever-out force of alternate cup designs reported in the literature have a wide range of differences in average force values [1]. As shown in Figures 1 and 2, the average push-out force is 1038 N and the average lever-out torque is 35.7 N·m. These values were measured under quasi-static, non-lubricated laboratory conditions. This wide range of values indicates that there is a wide diversity in cup designs and their corresponding shell/liner locking mechanisms. It is also important to recognize that some of the alternate designs incorporate a third locking component such as a metal wire retaining ring. Thus, even though they are called "two-piece" designs, they really are "three-piece" constructs. This could account for some of the wide range of test values.

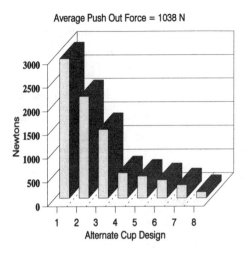

FIG. 1—Comparison of Push-Out Test Results

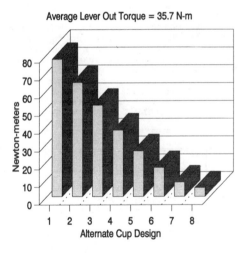

FIG. 2—Comparison of Lever-Out Test Results

This leads to the question of whether these values for each design would still be in the same range after moderate fatigue "break-in" cycling which would naturally occur *in vivo*. This question is essential to answer if there is to be confidence in the design integrity and if the proposed standard test methods are comprehensive in their design evaluation.

More importantly, there are reports in the literature of postoperative disassembly of two-piece acetabular components which should be carefully reviewed to determine if there is a correlation between fatigue cycling and loss of locking mechanism integrity between the metal shell and the UHMWPE liner [2-6]. If standard test methods included fatigue as a performance variable, could these early component failures have been avoided?

Materials and Methods

Tests for locking mechanism integrity were done in accordance with the ASTM Task Force F04.22.17 draft standard test methods for push-out and lever-out testing of modular acetabular cup systems (Draft Standard Test Method for Static Evaluation of Liner Locking Mechanism—Push-out Test, ASTM Task Force F04.22.17, 1994 and Draft Standard Test Method for Determination of the Lever-out Strength of Acetabular Shell/Liner Assemblies, ASTM Task Force F04.22.17, 1994). These methods are modifications from the published work of the Orthopaedic Research Laboratory of the Mt. Sinai Medical Center [1].

Specimens

Each of the acetabular cup liners and shells used as specimens for this study were taken from Wright Medical Technology (WMT) production inventory and are part of the WMT acetabular cup family. Sample size (n), or number of UHMWPE liners used for each type of test, are shown in Table 1. These polyethylene acetabular inserts (liners) accommodate 28 mm femoral heads, with corresponding acetabular shells. Relevant locking mechanism dimensions were characterized before testing to verify that the components met design specifications.

TABLE 1

Test	Pre-Fatigue	Post-Fatigue
Congruency	n = 3	n = 3
Push-Out	n = 7	n = 7
Lever-out	n = 7	n = 9

Shell/Liner Assembly

Each of the shell/liner combinations were assembled by loading with a 28 mm femoral head at a rate of 5.08 mm/minute (0.2 inches/minute). Assembly was accomplished with the use of an MTS 858 Biaxial Test System with an Interlaken DDC4000 servo-hydraulic controller.

Congruency

Six shell/liner combinations were assembled for evaluation of congruency between the components. Congruency measurements for "shell-liner gap" and "lock tab engagement" were made as shown in Figure 3. Three of these assemblies were sectioned for measurements of the congruency between the shell and liner without being subjected to fatigue loading. The three other assemblies were subjected to 2000 cycles of fatigue

loading in accordance with the test profile given below and then
sectioned after gait profile load cycling.

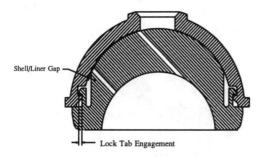

FIG. 3—Congruency Measurement Locations

Measurements of the six congruency specimens were then taken with a
Nikon Epiphot metallograph at 50x magnification to evaluate the
congruity or gap between the liner and shell and between the locking tab
and the shell. Three assemblies were measured without fatigue loading,
and an additional three assemblies were measured after fatigue loading.

Push-Out

Seven shell/liner assemblies were subjected to push-out tests without
fatigue test cycles, and seven other shell/liner assemblies were
subjected to push-out tests after the application of 2000 fatigue
cycles. Gait profile cycles were in accordance with the analysis done
by Komistek et al., as outlined in the section on fatigue [7].

Push-out tests were conducted by supporting the rim of the metal shell
and applying a constant displacement at a rate of 2.54 mm/minute (0.1
inches/minute) for both the unfatigued and fatigued shell/liner
assemblies. Displacement to cause disassembly of the liner was applied
by means of a 0.25 inch (6.35 mm) steel rod inserted through a hole in
the apex of the shell, as shown in Figure 4. For each test specimen,
the maximum recorded breakaway force was taken as the force required to
cause separation of the shell and liner. The percent change in push-out
force as a result of fatigue cycling was then evaluated.

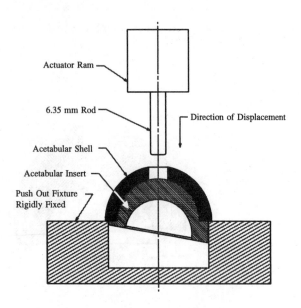

FIG. 4—Schematic of Push-out Test

Lever-out

Seven shell/liner assemblies were subjected to lever-out tests without fatigue test cycles, and nine other shell/liner assemblies were subjected to lever-out tests after the application of 2000 fatigue cycles. Gait profile cycles were also in accordance with the analysis done by Komistek et al., as outlined in the section on fatigue [7].

In preparation for lever-out tests, each metal shell was potted in a rectangular block of polymethylmethacrylate (PMMA) bone cement to allow adaptation to a standardized holding fixture. Lever-out tests were conducted by firmly clamping the PMMA block (that held the metal shell) into the holding fixture, as shown in Figure 5. A dislocation force was applied to each of the shell/liner assemblies (pre- and post-fatigue) through the use of a cylindrical lever bar inserted into a 6.35 mm (0.25 inch) hole that had been previously drilled into the I.D. of each plastic liner.

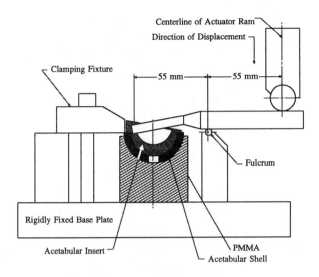

FIG. 5—Schematic of Lever-out Test

The lever bar was loaded at a rate of 50.8 mm/minute (2 inches/minute) about a fulcrum located at 55±3 mm from the drilled liner hole, as shown in Figure 5. Results were recorded as the load required to separate the liner from the shell. The percent change in lever-out force as a result of fatigue cycling was then evaluated.

Fatigue

Nineteen shell/liner assemblies were subjected to cyclic fatigue loading, three for congruency measurements, seven for push-out tests, and nine for lever-out tests. A multi-axis gait profile, simulating normal walking, was applied to each assembly for 2,000 cycles using an MTS 858 Multi-Axis Test System with Flextest servo-hydraulic control software. As shown in Figure 6, this dynamic loading is applied through a 28 mm femoral head. The gait profile included peak compression loading of about 2.5 times body weight (or about 1780 Newtons), rotation of approximately ± 5 degrees, and flexion of 0 to 30 degrees. The profile was derived from the work presented by Komistek et al. [7]. Further details of the gait profile are not presented here because the focus is on the effect of fatigue cycling and not the specifics of the fatigue gait cycle. Gait profile could be addressed by the standard methods.

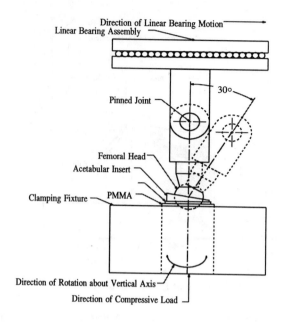

FIG. 6—Schematic of Fatigue Test Setup

The metal acetabular shell was potted in PMMA bone cement to enable it to be secured in the standardized test machine holding fixture. After fatigue cycling, each of the shell/liner assemblies was subjected to congruency, push-out, and lever-out tests as described above.

Results

Congruency

Measurements for congruency (or lack of gap) between the UHMWPE acetabular liner and the corresponding metal shell were made before and after fatigue cycling on two different assemblies, respectively. As shown in Figure 3, two locations were examined: (1) between the major mating spherical diameters of the liner and shell, and (2) between the UHMWPE locking tab of the liner and the adjacent locking surface of the metal shell.

Figure 7 shows the results of the measurements taken with the aid of the metallograph as the mean ± 1 standard deviation. It is interesting to note that the shell/liner gap at the spherical mating diameters *decreased* by an average of 34 percent after fatigue cycling. The lock tab engagement of the UHMWPE liner with the metal shell locking surface *increased* by an average of 28 percent. This means that the congruency between the liner and the shell actually improved in both areas of measurement.

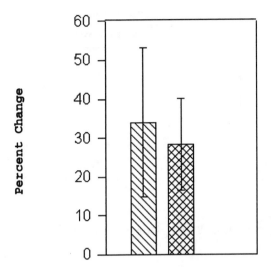

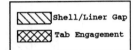

FIG. 7—Congruency Measurement Comparisons

Push-out

Push-out test results are shown in Figure 8, as the mean ± 1 standard deviation, for the fourteen specimens evaluated, seven without fatigue and seven after fatigue cycling. Comparison of the mean values shown in Figure 8 indicates that there was a 32.6 percent *increase* in the mean push-out value as the result of fatigue cycling. The difference in the mean values of the non-fatigued and the fatigued test samples was found to be statistically significant (P = 0.0026) as determined by the t-test. This implies that the locking integrity of this particular acetabular cup design, as measured by push-out tests, actually improved with moderate fatigue "break-in."

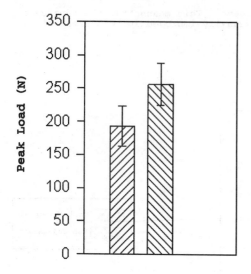

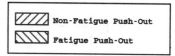

Non-Fatigue Push-Out

Fatigue Push-Out

FIG. 8—Push-Out Test Comparison

Lever-out

Lever-out test results are shown in Figure 9 as the mean ± 1 standard
deviation, for the disassembly force without fatigue compared to the
value with moderate fatigue cycling. There was a 6.3 percent *increase*
in the mean torque value to lever-out the liners from the shell after
fatigue cycling. However, this difference was not found to be
statistically significant (P = 0.6887) according to the t-test. More
test samples would be required to determine the actual statistical
effect, but this initial data implies that the lever-out torque would be
the same or slightly improved, according to the shift in the mean,
rather than decreased.

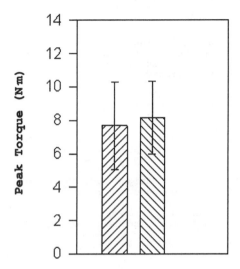

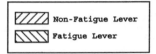

FIG. 9—Lever-Out Test Comparison

Discussion

This study has shown that moderate fatigue cycling improves the congruency and mean liner push-out strength for the particular acetabular cup design tested, and the mean lever-out strength was maintained. More specifically, in terms of congruity, the shell/liner gap was reduced by an average of 34 percent (a positive effect on the fit between the shell and liner), and the locking tab engagement was increased (or made more secure) by an average of 28 percent. For shell/liner locking integrity, the resulting mean of the push-out test values was 32.6 percent higher while the lever-out values were statistically similar both before and after fatigue cycling.

However, this result may not be universal for the variety of acetabular cup designs that are currently in existence [1]. It has been noted that there is a wide range of difference in the push-out and lever-out test values for the eight alternate cup designs tested in accordance with the proposed standard test methods. This clearly indicates distinct design differences and raises the question of whether each design would continue to have acceptable performance values after time *in vivo*.

Therefore, it is essential that standard test methods include an evaluation that takes into account the effect that could occur from fatigue. Only then can we have confidence that an effective comparison has been made between designs.

Conclusions and Recommendations

In conclusion, since there are reports in the literature of early disassembly of two-piece acetabular components *in vivo*, and since this study has shown an effect of fatigue for one particular design, fatigue cycling should be considered in design evaluations.

Since there is a wide range of performance for "alternate cup designs" and this study has shown that fatigue cycling can affect these values, there are two recommendations:

1.   Tests of the "alternate cup designs" should be redone to evaluate whether moderate fatigue cycling would have a positive or a negative effect on each of these designs.

2.   Consideration should be given to including fatigue cycling in the proposed standard test methods for push-out and lever-out tests.

ASTM Task Force F04.22.17 would be an appropriate forum for further discussions on this topic and for consideration of inclusion of fatigue cycling in the standard test methods.

Acknowledgement

The authors acknowledge the assistance of Mr. Michael Carroll of Mechanical Testing and Analysis, Inc., Memphis, TN and Dr. Warren Haggard of Wright Medical Technology, Inc.

References

[1]   Tradonsky, S., Postak, P. D., Froimson, A. I. and Greenwald, A. S., "A Comparison of the Disassociation Strength of Modular Acetabular Components," *Clinical Orthopaedics and Related Research*, No. 296, November 1993, pp. 154-160.

[2]   Beaver, R. J., Schemitsch, E. H., and Gross, A. E., "Disassembly of a One-Piece Metal-Backed Acetabular Component, A Case Report," *The Journal of Bone and Joint Surgery*, Vol. 73-B, No. 6, November 1991, pp. 908-910.

[3]   Bueche, M. J., Herzenberg, J. E., and Stubbs, B. T., "Dissociation of a Metal-backed Polyethylene Acetabular Component," *The Journal of Arthroplasty*, Vol. 4 No. 1, March 1989, pp. 39-41.

[4]   Kitziger, K. J., DeLee, J. C., and Evans, J. A., "Disassembly of a Modular Acetabular Component of a Total Hip-Replacement Arthroplasty," *The Journal of Bone and Joint Surgery*, Vol. 72-A, No. 4, April 1990, pp. 621-623.

[5]   Schmalzried, T. P., and Harris, W. H., "The Harris-Galante Porous-Coated Acetabular Component with Screw Fixation," *The Journal of Bone and Joint Surgery*, Vol. 74-A, No. 8, September 1992, pp. 1130-1139.

[6]   Star, M. J., Colwell, C. W., Donaldson, W. F., and Walker, R. H., "Dissociation of Modular Hip Arthroplasty Components After Dislocation, A Report of Three Cases at Differing Dissociation Levels," *Clinical Orthopaedics and Related Research*, No. 278, May 1992, pp. 111-115.

[7]   Komistek, R. D. et al., "Mathematical Model of the Human Lower Extremity," 13th Annual Southern Biomedical Engineering Conference, Washington, D.C., April 16-17, 1994.

Shilesh C. Jani[1], Willard L. Sauer[1], Terry W. McLean[2], Richard D. Lambert[1], and Paul Kovacs[3].

FRETTING CORROSION MECHANISMS AT MODULAR IMPLANT INTERFACES

REFERENCE: Jani, S. C., Sauer, W. L., McLean, T. W., Lambert, R. D., and Kovacs, P., **"Fretting Corrosion Mechanisms at Modular Implant Interfaces,"** *Modularity of Orthopedic Implants, ASTM STP 1301,* Donald E. Marlowe, Jack E. Parr, and Michael B. Mayor, Eds., American Society for Testing and Materials, 1997.

ABSTRACT: Modular connections have been commonly and successfully utilized in orthopaedic implant systems for the last 15 or so years, particularly at the head/neck junction in total hip arthroplasty (THA). However, recent retrieval studies have shown that some of the tapered junctions between femoral heads and stems in total hip arthoplasty can be prone to fretting corrosion, and may be a cause for concern in the longevity of implants. Fretting corrosion, which may release metallic products (particulate debris and ions) into the joint space, is a complex phenomenon in which the interplay between mechanically induced interfacial micromotion (fretting) and electrochemical corrosive activity play an important role, along with materials selection and processes. This suggests that interfacial fretting corrosion at modular implant interfaces can be significantly affected by the design variables of the modular junction. The working hypothesis of this study was that different designs of the modular head/stem combination of femoral hip prostheses exhibit different release of fretting corrosion metal products during fatigue testing used to simulate ten years of *in vivo* service. Three designs of femoral head (Co-Cr-Mo alloy) and stem (Ti-6Al-4V alloy) combinations were investigated in this study. The study included detailed taper metrology followed by environmental fatigue testing of the tapered junctions. The results of this study showed that important taper design differences do exist in the three constructs tested, and these differences manifested in different fretting corrosion behavior.

KEYWORDS: total hip arthroplasty, modular implants, taper fit, fretting corrosion, crevice corrosion.

[1]Senior Research Engineer, [2]Senior Research Technician, and [3]Manager of Surface Research, Orthopaedic Research and Development, Smith and Nephew Richards, Inc., 1450 Brooks Road, Memphis, TN 38116.

Modular connections are commonly employed in prosthetic implant constructs, particularly at the femoral head/neck interface in total hip arthroplasty (THA). Fretting corrosion at some modular interfaces, and release of metallic particulates and ions into the joint space have recently emerged as important causes for concern in total hip arthroplasty (THA), and have called into question the use of modular implants [1, 2]. The early femoral components in THA were one piece designs in which the femoral head and the stem were integral, and usually manufactured out of surgical grade 316L stainless steel. The introduction of ceramic femoral heads and Ti-6Al-4V alloy led to the use of modular components in which the femoral head and the stem were mated, either intraoperatively or by the manufacturer, via a Morse cone taper. This modularity affords several tangible advantages for the manufacturer, and the surgical team as listed below:

1. the surgical team is better able to match intraoperatively the patient anatomy,
2. the components are tailored for optimum function. For instance Ti-6Al-4V alloy is used for the stems due to its biocompatibility and lower stiffness, while Co-Cr-Mo alloy, and ceramic alumina and zirconia are used for the femoral heads due to their superior tribological properties, and
3. the inventory required to serve the range of patient anatomic variability is reduced.

Notwithstanding these advantages, the modular connections present a potential for in vivo dissociation, and corrosion. Service dissociation of the head from the stem has been reported for some modular implants [3, 4]. The potential for crevice and galvanic corrosion occurring at the dissimilar metal head/neck interface was considered and investigated at the onset of the use of modularity. Using mechanically static conditions (unloaded), investigators found that mating similar and dissimilar alloys, e.g., Co-Cr-Mo/Co-Cr-Mo, Ti-6Al-4V/Ti-6Al-4V, and Co-Cr-Mo/Ti-6Al-4V did not significantly influence the electrochemical corrosive behavior of either component of the couple [5, 6]. This behavior was attributed to the ability of the alloys to form passive films on the surfaces, and the tenacity of these passive films under crevice and galvanic coupled conditions.

Incidence of corrosion found at revision surgery at the tapered junctions were reported in the early 1990's [7, 8]. Initially, the reports seemed to indicate that corrosion at the tapered interface was exclusive to components with mixed alloy couples, i.e., Ti-6Al-4V stem/Co-Cr-Mo head combinations, and that such mixed alloy couples were inherently susceptible to corrosion [7]. Further retrieval studies showed that similar alloy couples of Co-Cr-Mo/Co-Cr-Mo can also exhibit in vivo corrosion [8, 9], while some couples of mixed Ti-6Al-4V stem/Co-Cr-Mo head showed no corrosion [10].

These retrieval studies suggest that the corrosion observed must result from a complex set of mechano-electrochemical activities, which include interfacial stresses, (micro) motion, crevice geometries, and material conditions. It is now recognized that this phenomenon is fretting accelerated crevice corrosion [9, 11]. Various research groups have strived to identify the salient features of fretting corrosion via *in vitro* testing [12, 13]. Since both mechanical fretting, and electrochemical corrosion activity together play a pivotal role, it stands to reason that design of the femoral component and of the tapered junction would influence the fretting corrosion phenomena, as discussed below.

Taper Design Variables

A typical modular femoral component is shown schematically in Figure 1, along with geometric design variables. The important design variables are discussed in detail below, along with their impact on the fretting corrosion performance:

- **Medial-Lateral Offset.** The medial-lateral (M-L) offset is an important design variable, in that it needs to be matched to the patient for restoration of joint biomechanics. The mechanical loads are transferred through the head center to the distal aspect of the femur via the cantilever formed by the neck region of the femoral component. The longer the M-L offset, the higher will be the bending loads (and strains) at the tapered neck. All other parameters being equal, the M-L offset will control the amount of relative motion between the head and the stem at the tapered junction, and hence the tendency for fretting.

- **Neck Length.** The neck length (NL) of the design plays an important role in restoring the leg length of the patient. For a given femoral stem, the neck length is controlled via the use of heads with different female taper depths. The longer the neck length, the longer will be the M-L offset.

- **Taper Diameter.** The taper diameter (Ø) is defined at a particular reference or gage point along the length of the taper. The importance of the diameter is multi-fold; the diameter dictates the static and fatigue strength, it influences the range of motion of the hip prosthesis, and the bending stresses and strains along the taper. From basic mechanics, the bending stresses and strains in a circular cross-section beam in cantilever bending increase inversely with the third power of the diameter.

- **Included Angle.** The included angle (α) for the head/neck tapers are typically in the 4 to 7 degree range.

- **Angle Mismatch.** The angle mismatch (Δα) is defined as the difference between the included angles of the head taper and the neck taper. In Figure 1, the head taper angle is greater than the neck taper angle (positive mismatch). When the neck taper angle is greater than the head taper angle the mismatch would be negative.

Manufacturers strive to design femoral components to best accommodate the ranges in each of these variables encountered in the human population. Femoral components are designed such that these variables change either independent of each other, or depending on each other. For instance, in some designs the M-L offset is controlled only via the choice of neck length (of the head) for all stem sizes, while in other designs, the M-L offset varies with

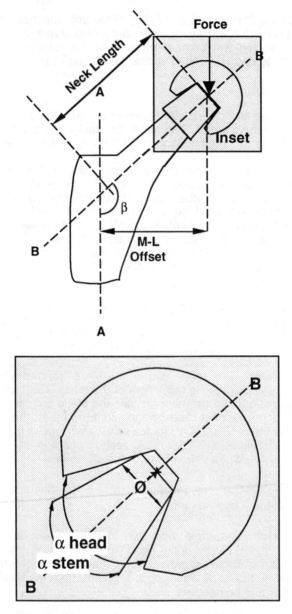

Figure 1--Schematic illustrations of the proximal aspect of the femoral head and stem construct. The design variables which impact the fretting corrosion behavior of the modular junction are identified, and expanded upon in the text.

the neck length and the size (stem length, distal diameter, etc.) of the stem. The importance of these design variables is that they will dictate the choice of the stem/head combination, and therefore may influence the fretting corrosion behavior.

OBJECTIVE

The working hypothesis of the present study was that different modular femoral hip components with different taper designs exhibit different fretting corrosion behavior. The objective of the study was to subject three different designs of femoral hip stems and heads to detailed metrological analyses to determine the taper design characteristics, followed by fatigue testing of the individual constructs to determine the extent of fretting corrosion damage as a function of design variables.

MATERIALS AND METHODS

Materials

Three combinations of head (Co-Cr-Mo alloy) and stem (Ti-6Al-4V alloy) of different design were used in this study to test the hypothesis that fretting corrosion is design dependent. The different designs were designated A, B and C. The nominal diameters were 14.33 mm for design A, and 10.26 mm for designs B and C.

The Co-Cr-Mo alloy heads utilized in this study were 28 mm diameter for all designs tested. Furthermore, the head taper depth (neck length) for all three designs were equivalent (within 1 mm). This ensured that it was the design of the tapered junction that was tested, and not the effect of neck length. The Ti-6Al-4V alloy porous coated hip stems used in this study were chosen such that for all designs the M-L offset was exactly the same at 38 mm. This aspect of the experimental method ensured that the mechanical bending moment was the same for all three designs.

Pre-Test Taper Characterization

Prior to fatigue testing, all tapers were fully metrologically characterized. Taper included angles and taper conicity were measured on a coordinate measuring machine (CMM), while stylus profilometry was utilized for determining taper roughness (R_a), and straightness. Taper angle mismatch was determined from the included angle data. Taper straightness is a measure of how straight the profile of the taper is at along a line traced by the plane that goes through the axial center of the taper. Taper conicity is a measure of the roundness of the circumference formed by a plane perpendicular to the axis of the taper. The higher these values, the less straight and less conical is the taper.

Assembly and Fatigue Testing

The tapers were thoroughly cleaned and degreased prior to assembly and testing. The fatigue testing was conducted with the hip stems fully potted to the osteotomy line with bone cement. The heads were assembled to the potted stems by applying an axial load of 2003 N (450 lbf). After assembly, the head/neck region was encapsulated with tygon tubing and sealed on both ends with silicone elastomer. After the elastomer had cured, approximately 10 ml of Lactated Ringer's Irrigation (McGaw, Inc., Irvine, CA) was injected into the encapsulated tapered interface with a syringe. The test set up is shown schematically in Figure 2. Fatigue testing was conducted on close-looped

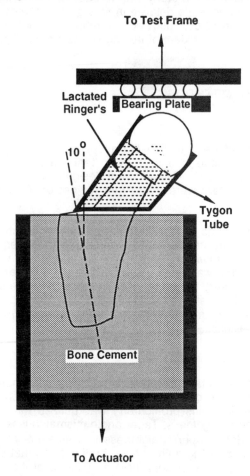

Figure 2--Schematic illustration of the fatigue test set up, including the Lactated Ringer's Irrigation in the encapsulated taper region. The stems were potted to the osteotomy line with bone cement.

servo hydraulic testing machines, with the components oriented 10 degrees laterally and 10 degrees in the anterior-posterior direction. Fatigue testing was conducted for 10 million cycles at a compressive load range of 330 N to 3303 N (74 lbf to 742 lbf) and a frequency of 10 Hz.

Post-Fatigue Testing

After completion of 10 million loading cycles, the Ringer's solution was withdrawn with a syringe. 10 ml of double dionized (DI) water was injected into the encapsulated taper junction, and withdrawn after agitation. Each test solution was diluted with DI water to yield a sample of 50 ml. One ml of 50/50 mixture of nitric and hydrofluoric acids were added to each test sample to digest any solid metallic particulates. The test samples were then sent to a commercial laboratory (Teledyne Wah Chang Albany Analytical Services, Albany, OR) for analyses of cobalt, chromium and titanium content by direct coupled plasma optical emission spectroscopy (DCP-OES).

Each test assembly was then disassembled on a servo hydraulic test frame, and the axial force to distract was recorded.

RESULTS

All mean measured pre-test taper measurements are shown in Table 1. The standard deviations of the measurement are shown in parenthesis following the mean values.

TABLE 1--Mean (s.d.) pre-test characteristics of the tapers

	DESIGN A n = 3		DESIGN B n = 3		DESIGN C n = 3	
	Head	Stem	Head	Stem	Head	Stem
Nominal Diameter (mm)	14.33		10.26		10.26	
Straightness (μm)	1.85 (0.64)	1.1 (1.1)	3.37 (1.97)	10.80 (2.6)	1.20 (0.13)	2.29 (0.56)
Conicity (μm)	8.20 (0.66)	8.64 (0.61)	23.54 (14.03)	11.6 (3.8)	49.53 (4.14)	9.07 (0.79)
Roughness (μm)	0.36 (0.07)	2.05 (0.26)	0.96 (0.37)	0.62 (0.1)	0.33 (0.14)	0.41 (0.04)
Included Angle (°)	5.715 (0.004)	5.659 (0.014)	5.762 (0.008)	5.639 (0.012)	5.733 (0.084)	5.979 (0.005)
Mismatch (°)	0.06 (0.016)		0.12 (0.019)		− 0.25 (0.087)	

The above table clearly shows that the three designs had different taper metrology. For the pairs of groups within the three groups tested, statistical significance ($p < 0.05$, paired t-test) was established for the following:

• The nominal taper diameter was larger for group A than groups B and C, and equal for groups B and C.
• Stem tapers in groups A and C were straighter than in group B.
• The head tapers in group A were more conical than in groups B and C. The head tapers in group B were more conical than in group C.
• Head tapers in group B were rougher than in groups A and C.
• Stem tapers in group A were rougher than in groups B and C.
• The taper angle mismatch was greater in group C than in groups A and C, and was greater in group C than group B.

The other differences were not statistically significant. The taper angle and mismatch results indicate that on axial assembly, the initial contact takes place proximally (head angle > stem angle) in designs A and B, while initial contact in design C is distal (stem angle > head angle).

The axial distraction forces to release the head from the stem, and the metal release data for the three designs tested are shown in Table 2. In all designs, the highest metal levels were of cobalt, followed by chromium. Design A exhibited the lowest total metal release, followed by design B, and design C. Design B released approximately ten times more metal than design A, while design C released approximately 20 times more metal than design A. These differences were statistically significant. The titanium levels of all three test solutions extracted from design A, and two of the three test solutions extracted from design C were below the detection limit for DCP-OES (0.05 µg/ml). Conversely, all three tests of design B showed detectable titanium levels. It is interesting to note that the ratio of cobalt to chromium released from the tapers during fatigue testing was 3.3, 2.9, and 3.4 for design A, B and C respectively, while the same ratio in the Co-Cr-Mo alloy (ASTM F 75 and F 799) is approximately 2.2.

TABLE 2--<u>Mean (s.d.) distraction forces, and metal released</u>

	DESIGN A n = 3	DESIGN B n = 3	DESIGN C n = 3
Distraction Force (N)	4224 (2137)	4273 (2753)	2217 (307)
Cobalt (µg)	25 (13)	255 (58)	566 (148)
Chromium (µg)	7.5 (4)	88 (23)	165 (36)
Titanium (µg)	<2.5	44 (6)	32 (54)[*]
Total Metal (µg)	32.5	387	763

[*]Only one test solution for design C showed detectable titanium for the DCP-OES technique (0.05 µg/ml).

The distraction forces to separate the head/neck assemblies did not exhibit statistically different results for the three designs tested. Visual examination of the tapers showed that design A had undergone no visible signs of fretting or corrosion on either the stem or the head tapers. Design C, on the other hand showed the most significant extent of taper surface damage, with the damage predominantly localized at the distal-medial aspect, close to the mouth of the taper interface. Brown-green deposits were found on all stem and head tapers of design C. Design B showed intermediate level of visible damage, with the damage localized to the proximal rim region in two out of three tests. The remaining test sample in design B showed damage at the mid-taper region along the medial aspect. The medial surfaces of the post-test stem tapers are shown macroscopically in Figures 3a-c for designs A, B, and C respectively.

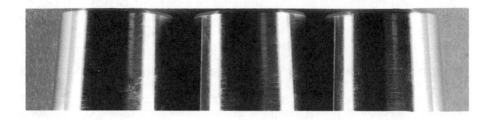

(a) Design A

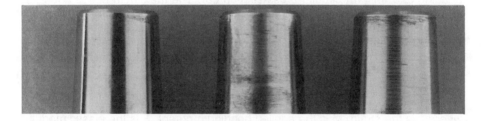

(b) Design B

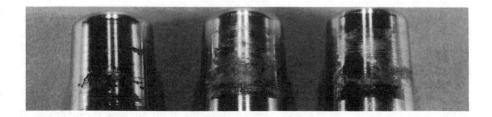

(c) Design C

Figure 3--Macrophotographs of the medial engagement regions of stem tapers after testing.

DISCUSSION

The results of this study have shown that different tapers exhibit different metrological characteristics, and these differences are manifested in varying fretting corrosion behavior. The taper metrology variations may result from different designs and/or from quality control (QC) of taper surfaces. Furthermore, the ratios of cobalt to chromium released from the tapers were greater than the cobalt to chromium ratio in the base Co-Cr-Mo alloy, suggesting that cobalt was selectively depleted from the head tapers. This selective depletion of cobalt implies that corrosion played an important role in the metal release process, together with mechanical fretting. The influence of taper design and QC on fretting corrosion is discussed in detail below.

<u>Taper Diameter</u>

The nominal taper diameter for design A was 14.33 mm, while for designs B and C was approximately 10.26 mm. The taper diameter has important implications in the fretting corrosion behavior, primarily because it controls the bending stresses and strains along the length of the taper. During cyclic loading of the taper, the higher the strain range, the higher will be the relative micromotion at the point of engagement between the stem and head tapers. The relative effect of different diameters may be approximated from simple bending of a uniform circular cross-section bar. The maximum stress and strain at a given distance from the point of fixture will occur at the outer diameter, with the opposite ends being in tension and compression, and is given by the following relationship:

$$\varepsilon_{max} = \frac{4 \ M}{E \ \pi \ r^3} \tag{1}$$

where ε is the strain, M is the applied bending moment, E is the elastic modulus, and r is the radius of the beam. This shows that the maximum stress and strain are inversely related to the third power of the beam radius (or diameter). Therefore, the micromotion caused by bending of the stem taper will also be a function of the diameter of the taper; the smaller the taper diameter, the larger the relative micromotion. For the three designs tested in this study, the ratio of the third powers of the diameters of A (Ø = 14.33 mm) and B and C (Ø = 10.26 mm) was calculated to be 2.72. This indicates that the stem tapers in designs B and C will exhibit micromotion due to bending to an extent at least twice as design A, and may therefore show greater fretting corrosion. Although designs B and C did exhibit greater fretting corrosion metal release than design A, the ratios of metal release did not follow the magnitude predicted by the diameters. If the taper diameter was the sole controlling factor, then designs B and C would be expected to undergo equivalent extent of fretting corrosion, which was not borne out in this study. This indicates that bending (and therefore taper diameter) alone may not be responsible for the differences in metal release.

Taper Angle Mismatch

The head taper angles were always greater than the stem taper angles in designs A and B, while in design C, the head tapers angles were always lesser than the stem taper angles. This difference may have important implications in the fretting corrosion behavior, as illustrated in Figure 4. It is important to note here that even in cases where the bending strains are infinitesimally small (infinite elastic modulus), the head and stem tapers at the rim of engagement will undergo relative motion from the rocking of the head. This rocking motion will depend on the moment arm formed by the distance between the center of the head (the point through which load is transmitted) and the rim of contact, and the frictional resistance forces acting at contact. The initial engagement of the stem and head tapers in designs A and B will occur at the proximal region (throat contact), while for design C the initial engagement will occur at the distal region (mouth contact). As shown in Figure 4, the distance between the center of the head (marked "X" in Figure 4) and the rim of contact in design C is greater than in designs A and B. This implies that moment arms acting at both medial (M_M) and lateral (M_L) contact points will be higher in design C than in designs A and B. Design C will therefore undergo greater impingement of the head at the medial aspect of the stem taper, and correspondingly higher relative sliding motion at the lateral aspect. This rocking motion of the head would be minimized if there existed a perfect fit between the head and stem tapers, i.e., if the angle mismatch was zero. In the present study, design C was found to have a greater magnitude of mismatch than designs A and B, and design B had greater mismatch than design A.

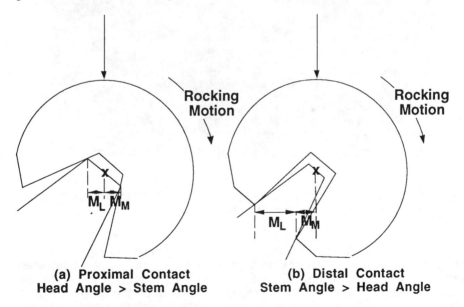

(a) Proximal Contact
Head Angle > Stem Angle

(b) Distal Contact
Stem Angle > Head Angle

Figure 4--A schematic illustration of the influence of the sign of taper angle mismatch between the head and stem.

Another implication of proximal versus distal contact, is that the geometry of the crevices formed will be different. The crevice in designs A and B will be more open to the joint fluids outside the taper, and therefore more amenable for physical and diffusional transport of oxygen, which in turn would allow for re-passivation of any localized areas damaged by fretting. The crevice in design C, on the other hand is closed to the external joint fluids. However, any fluid that may have seeped into the crevice by wicking (capillarity) during active ambulation will remain enclosed within the crevice during the non-ambulatory phase of the patient, and cause significant crevice corrosion. This may have been a major contributory factor in the different fretting corrosion behavior between the three designs tested. During the fatigue tests, bubbles were observed emerging at the medial aspect of the mouth of the taper in design C, as shown in Figure 5, while none were observed in designs A and B. Although not verified experimentally, these bubbles may be hydrogen gas from corrosion occurring within the crevices, or air released from the tapers in design C.

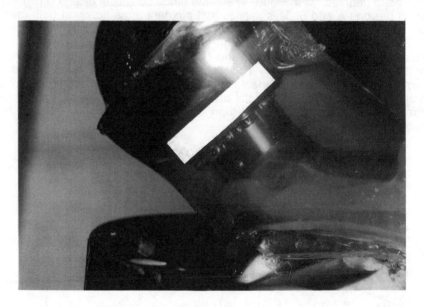

Figure 5--Bubbles observed emanating from the medial mouth region during fatigue testing of a head/stem construct of design C.

From the preceding discussion, the combination of greater rocking motion and stagnated crevices in designs with distal contact may have contributed significantly to the 20 times difference in the fretting corrosion metal release between designs A and C. While rocking of the head on the stem may have contributed to the magnitude of total metal release in designs A and B, the ten times difference between them probably cannot be attributed all to rocking because both of these designs have proximal contact. The larger angular mismatch in design B than design A may have contributed to a measurable extent.

Taper Straightness, Conicity and Roughness

Taper straightness and conicity are clearly quality control parameters. For ideal performance, the tapers should be as straight, and as-conical in shape as the manufacturing practices allow. Significant deviations from straight and conical shape will affect where, along the tapers, contact between the head and the stem takes place, and therefore the tendency for fretting and crevice corrosion. No parametric studies to investigate the contribution of taper straightness and conicity have been reported to date, and therefore the significance of these parameters in the magnitude of fretting corrosion cannot be estimated. However, as shown in the Results section, the stem straightness, and the head conicity in group A were better than groups B and C. These differences may have contributed to the different fretting corrosion behavior.

The head roughness values were equivalent for the three designs. The mean stem roughness, however, was greater for design A than designs B and C. The coarser, and deeper machined grooves in design A may allow for more uniform and predictable contact between the stem and head tapers because the peaks of the grooves would more easily deform to conform to the geometry of the head on contact.

The preceding discussion has argued that taper design and QC variables can have a significant influence on the fretting corrosion behavior of modular taper interfaces. Mechano-electrochemical mechanisms which would play out due to design and QC variable differences, and therefore control the fretting corrosion behavior were postulated. The testing conducted during this study has shown that fretting corrosion of the nature observed in some clinical retrievals can be duplicated in the laboratory, and can be used to guide taper design optimization processes.

Clinical Perspective Of Taper Fretting Corrosion

The metal release data generated in this study should be put into proper clinical perspective. In a recent study [14] it was demonstrated that periprosthetic tissue around hip implants that showed visible (macroscopic) signs of corrosion contained corrosion products released from the taper. This study also showed that the amount of serum cobalt and urine chromium at the time of revision surgery was elevated in patients whose implants showed moderate to severe taper corrosion compared to patients whose implants showed none to mild taper corrosion. These findings suggest that taper corrosion increases the metallic burden, particularly cobalt and chromium from the femoral head. It is well known that there exist multiple interfaces in a typical total joint replacement, all of which contribute to the total burden of metallic particles and ions released into the host environment. Of all the interfaces, the only one designed for motion is, of course, the articulating interface, which typically involves the articulation of Co-Cr-Mo alloy against ultra high molecular weight polyethylene (UHMWPE).

This articulation will release significant quantities of polyethylene particles, and Co-Cr-Mo in ionic and particulate form [15], even when the metallic implant is monolithic (non-modular). The release of metallic fretting corrosion products from taper interfaces should be compared to these quantities of Co-Cr-Mo wear products released from articulation. Simple laboratory testing of Co-Cr-Mo heads articulating against UHMWPE liners has shown that significant quantities of cobalt can be released [16], and when the data is extrapolated to 10 million cycles, the cobalt and chromium release from articulation alone (926 and 289 µg respectively) can be higher than that released by design C tested in this study, and much greater than either design A or B. This indicates that although tapers in modular implants may be an additional source of metallic wear products, they can be designed such that the contribution is minuscule compared to metal released from the articulating surface.

CONCLUSIONS

This investigation showed that the head and stem tapers in modular femoral hip components exhibit different design and quality control (QC) variables. Fretting corrosion testing of three different designs showed that metal release from the tapers can vary from design to design by well over an order of magnitude. Parametric studies to determine the relative influence of all taper design and QC variables are encouraged.

REFERENCES

[1] Urban, R. M., Jacobs, J. J., Gilbert, J. L., and Galante, J. O., "Migration of Corrosion Products from Modular Hip Prostheses: Particle Microanalyses and Histopathological Findings", The Journal of Bone and Joint Surgery, Vol. 76-A, No. 9, September 1994, pp 1345-1359.

[2] Salvati, E. A., Moderator, The Hip Society, Twenty-Third Open Scientific Meeting, Orlando, FL., February 1995.

[3] Barrack, R. L., Burke, D. W., Cook, S. D., Skinner, H. B., and Harris, W. H., "Complications related to Modularity of Total Hip Components", The Journal of Bone and Joint Surgery, Vol. 75-B, No. 5, September 1993, pp 688-692.

[4] Star, M. J., Colwell, C. W., Donaldson, W. F., and Walker, R. H., "Dissociation of Modular Hip Arthoplasty Components After Dislocation: A Report of Three Cases at Differing Dissociation Levels", Clinical Orthopaedics and Related Research, No. 278, May 1992, pp 111-115.

[5] Rostoker, W., Pretzel, C. W., and Galante, J. O., "Couple Corrosion Among Alloys for Skeletal Prostheses", Journal of Biomedical Materials Research, Vol. 8, 1974, pp 407-419.

[6]   Mears, D. C., "The Use of Dissimilar Metals in Surgery", Journal of Biomedical Materials Research, Vol. 6, 1975, pp 133-148.

[7]   Collier, J. P., Surprenant, V. A., Jensen, R. E., and Mayor, M. B., "Corrosion at the Interface of Cobalt-Alloy Heads on Titanium-Alloy Stems", Clinical Orthopaedics and Related Research, No. 271, October 1991, pp 305-312.

[8]   Mathiesen, E. B., Lindgren, J. U., Blomgren, G. A., and Reinholt, F. P., "Corrosion of Modular Hip Prostheses", The Journal of Bone and Joint Surgery, Vol. 73-B, No. 4, July 1991, pp 569-575.

[9]   Gilbert, J. L., Buckley, C. A., and Jacobs, J. J., "In Vivo Corrosion of Modular Hip Prosthesis Components in Mixed and Similar Metal Combinations. The Effect of Crevice, Stress, Motion, and Alloy Coupling", Journal of Biomedical Materials Research, Vol. 27, 1993, pp 1533-1544.

[10]   Sauer, W. A., Kovacs, P., Beals, N., and Cuckler, J., "Corrosion at Head/Taper Interfaces: A 3-5 Year Follow-Up of Modular Head/Ti-6Al-4V Femoral Stem Prostheses", Implant Retrieval Symposium Transactions, Society of Biomaterials, St. Charles, IL., September 1992, p 56.

[11]   Brown, S. A., Flemming, C. A. C., Kawalec, J. S., Placko, H. E., Vassaux, C., Merritt, K., Payer, J. H., and Kraay, M. J., "Fretting Corrosion Accelerates Crevice Corrosion of Modular Hip Tapers", Journal of Applied Biomaterials, Vol. 6, 1995, pp 19-26.

[12]   Bhambri, S., and Gilbertson, L., "Accelerated In Vitro Testing of Modular Joints to Simulate In Vivo Performance", 21st Annual Meeting Transactions, Society of Biomaterials, San Francisco, CA., March 1995, p 392.

[13]   Gilbert, J. L., Buckley, C. A., Jacobs, J. J., and Lautenschlager, E. P, "In Vitro Mechanical-Electrochemical Testing of the Fretting Corrosion Process in Modular Femoral Tapers", 41st Annual Meeting Transactions, Orthopaedic Research Society, Orlando, FL., February 1995, Vol. 20 - Section 1, p 240.\

[14]   Jacobs, J. J., Urban, R. M., Gilbert, J. L., Skipor, A. K., Black, J., Jasty, M., and Galante, J. O., "Local and Distant Products From Modularity", Clinical Orthopaedics and Related Research, No. 319, October 1995, pp 94-105.

[15]   Black, J., "Does Corrosion Matter", Editorial, The Journal of Bone and Joint Surgery, Vol. 70-B, No. 4, August 1988, pp 517-520.

[16]   Kovacs, P., and Davidson, J. A., "Fundamental Aspects of Wear-Accelerated Metal Ion Release: Metallic Versus Ceramic Bearing Surfaces", 38th Annual Meeting Transactions, Orthopaedic Research Society, Washington, D.C., February 1992, Vol. 17 - Section 2, p 349.

Christine S. Heim,[1] Paul D. Postak,[1] and A. Seth Greenwald[1]

FEMORAL STEM FATIGUE CHARACTERISTICS OF MODULAR HIP DE-
SIGNS

REFERENCE: Heim, C. S., Postak, P. D., and Greenwald, A. S., "**Femoral Stem Fatigue Characteristics of Modular Hip Designs**," Modularity of Orthopedic Implants, ASTM STP 1301, Donald E. Marlowe, Jack E. Parr, and Michael B. Mayor, Eds., American Society for Testing and Materials, 1997.

ABSTRACT: Modularity in total hip arthroplasty design has received increased citation in the literature. Clinical concerns in the application of these systems include structural compromise at metal-metal interconnections due to cyclic microdisplacements. A laboratory fatigue test method, incorporating proximal support was developed and utilized to determine performance characteristics for these systems. Structural fatigue curves for four modular systems currently in clinical use were obtained and compared to anticipated in vivo service loading conditions for the normal hip. The structural fatigue strength of these designs was at least 1.3 times the anticipated service load. The results demonstrate that the in vivo structural integrity of these systems should not be compromised by the presence of metal-metal interconnections.

KEYWORDS: modular hip design, fatigue characteristics, structural fatigue curve, proximal fatigue stem testing, and intercomponent fretting characteristics.

NOMENCLATURE

Anteversion - an axial rotation resulting in anterior advancement of the femoral head.

Endurance limit - the maximum cyclic load an implant system can sustain and theoretically never fail.

Implant service load - the maximum in vivo dynamic load on the hip during walking gait.

[1]Engineering Associate, Engineering Associate and Director, respectively, Orthopaedic Research Laboratories, Mt. Sinai Medical Center, One Mt. Sinai Dr, Cleveland, OH 44106.

Margin of safety - the difference between the endurance limit and the implant service load.

Neck offset or moment arm - the distance between the central axis of the distal stem and the location of load application on the femoral head.

Structural fatigue curve - a plot displaying applied cyclic load versus the log number of cycles.

INTRODUCTION

Modularity in total hip arthroplasty design is an evolving concept that is receiving increased citation in the clinical literature. The advantages of these systems include off the shelf flexibility for customizing proximal and distal canal filling as well as accommodating difficult situations of femoral deformity and bone loss [1-4]. Clinical concerns in the application of these modular hip designs include maintenance of anatomical stability within the femoral canal, structural compromise at metal-metal interconnections due to cyclic microdisplacements (fretting), corrosion of the femoral head/neck taper, intercomponent dislocation and an increased potential for metallic wear debris generation [5-15].

Because of the increasing clinical utilization of proximally supported stems the development of test methods which demonstrate structural safety under these loading conditions is required. Current International Standards Organization guidelines (Determination of Properties of Stemmed Femoral Components with Application of Torsion, ISO 7206-4) specify distal fixation for the fatigue testing of femoral stems. These methods are inadequate for the evaluation of composite, modular and monolithic systems which rely on proximal support for stability and load carriage *in vivo*.

This paper presents a laboratory fatigue method utilizing proximal support to evaluate four contemporary modular femoral stem designs and determine their structural integrity in terms of fatigue behavior.

TESTING METHODOLOGY

The test assembly was configured to allow load transmission through a proximally fixed femoral stem design with simple distal support (Fig. 1). This apparatus facilitated component alignment insuring reproducible load application. A closed loop servo hydraulic Materials Testing System (MTS Corporation, Eden Prairie, MN) was utilized for the application of controlled loads.

The proximal portion of each stem was rigidly fixed in acrylic across all porous coated surfaces to simulate optimal anticipated bone contact. The components were mounted with an anterior-posterior (A-P) rotational axis that passed through the intersection of the neck axis and the long axis of the stem in neutral anteversion. A sinusoidal loading sequence was applied parallel to the stem through the femoral head. A simple distal support counters the loading moment about the A-P axis, allowing maximum bending stresses to occur on the lateral side of the component. All testing was performed in an air environment at frequencies ranging from 10 to 15 Hz.

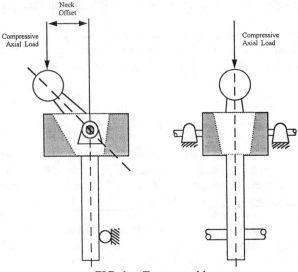

FIG. 1 -- Test assembly.

Multiple femoral stem systems of each design were evaluated at compressive sinusoidal load profiles (10% to 100% load), one profile per stem , until failure or 10 million cycles. The initial peak test load was 80% of the maximum bending stress calculated for a Ti-6Al-4V cantilever beam with the approximate dimensions of the particular femoral stem design. Based on the number of cycles to failure the peak load for each subsequent stem was varied in an attempt to attain the maximum load the design could support to 10 million cycles without failure. This resulted in a relatively unique sequence of peak load for each femoral stem design. The number of cycles and peak load for each femoral stem system were plotted on a semi-log scale to create a structural fatigue curve particular to each implant design [16-18].

MATERIALS

IMPACT Modular Hip System

The IMPACT Modular Hip System (Biomet, Inc., Warsaw, IN) offers modularity through a variety of femoral heads, metaphyseal segments and diaphyseal components (Fig. 2). A compression fit taper is utilized at the femoral head/neck and metaphyseal/diaphyseal component junctions and an auxiliary locking screw further secures the metaphyseal and diaphyseal components. The diaphyseal component contains distal cutting flutes and a coronal slot configuration. In this evaluation, the metaphyseal/diaphyseal tapered connection represents the location with the highest potential for crack initiation due to the high magnitude of the bending stresses on the lateral side of the component and the probability of fretting within the taper. The femoral stem evaluated was collarless and 151 mm in length with a 15 mm distal diameter. Medium-sized metaphyseal segments, 6.35 mm segment locking screws and 32 +0 mm femoral heads were also utilized in the evaluation of this design. All of the components were Ti-6Al-4V except the femoral head which was cobalt-chromium-molybdenum alloy. The resulting neck offset for this system was 37.5 mm.

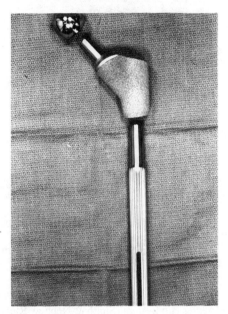

FIG. 2 -- IMPACT Modular Hip System.

INFINITY Modular Hip System

The INFINITY Modular Hip System (Wright Medical Technology, Inc., Arlington, TN) provides modularity through a variety of femoral heads, trochanteric modules and distal stems (Fig. 3). A compression fit taper is utilized at the femoral head/neck and trochanteric/stem component junctions. The taper between the trochanteric module and the distal stem is angled at 27 degrees relative to the vertical axis of the stem. The distal stem contains grooves. In this evaluation, the trochanteric/stem tapered connection represents the location with the highest potential for crack initiation due to the high magnitude of the bending stresses on the lateral side of the component and the probability of fretting within the taper. The femoral stem evaluated had a collar and was 150 mm in length with a 14 mm distal diameter. Medium-sized, porous coated trochanteric modules and 32 +0 mm femoral heads were also utilized in the evaluation of this design. All of the components were Ti-6Al-4V except the femoral head which was cobalt-chromium-molybdenum alloy. The resulting neck offset for this design was 46 mm.

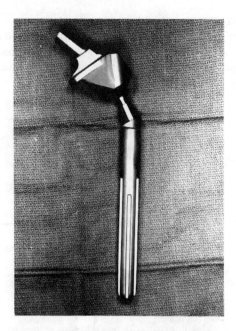

FIG. 3 -- INFINITY Modular Hip System.

RMHS Modular Hip System

The RMHS Modular Hip System (Smith & Nephew Richards, Memphis, TN) offers modularity through a variety of femoral heads, femoral stems, augmentation pads, distal sleeves and femoral neck extenders (Fig. 4). A compression fit taper is utilized at the femoral head/neck extender/femoral neck and stem/distal sleeve junctions. The augmentation pads are attached to the femoral stem through a compression fit lock key mechanism. In this evaluation, the proximal, lateral porous coated region represents the location with the highest potential for crack initiation due to the high magnitude of the bending stresses on the lateral side of the component and the stress riser effect associated with the porous bead sintering process. The femoral stem evaluated was collarless and 145 mm in length with a 12 mm distal diameter. The posterior, porous coated proximal augmentation pad was flush with the surface of the stem and a +6 mm porous coated, proximal augmentation pad was utilized on the anterior side of the stem. Fifteen millimeter diameter distal sleeves, +12 mm neck trunnion extenders and 32 + 8 mm femoral heads were also utilized in the evaluation of this design. All of the components were Ti-6Al-4V except the femoral head which was cobalt-chromium-molybdenum alloy. The resulting neck offset for this design was 50 mm.

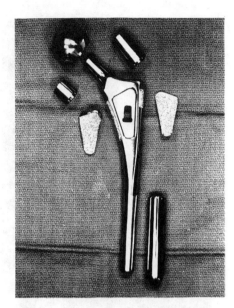

FIG. 4 -- RMHS Modular Hip System.

S-ROM Modular Hip System

The S-ROM Modular Hip System (Joint Medical Products Corporation, Stamford, CT) offers modularity through a variety of femoral heads, femoral stems and proximal sleeves (Fig. 5). A compression fit taper is utilized between the femoral head/neck and femoral stem/sleeve junctions. The stem contains distal cutting flutes and a coronal slot configuration. In this evaluation, the femoral stem/sleeve tapered connection represents the location with the highest potential for crack initiation due to the high magnitude of the bending stresses on the lateral side of the component and the probability of fretting within the taper. The femoral stem was lateralized +8 mm in the proximal region, collarless and 160 mm in length with a 13 mm distal diameter. Medium-sized, porous coated proximal sleeves and 28 +6 mm femoral heads were also utilized in the evaluation of this design. All of the components were Ti-6Al-4V except the femoral head which was cobalt-chromium-molybdenum alloy. The resulting neck offset for this design was 44 mm.

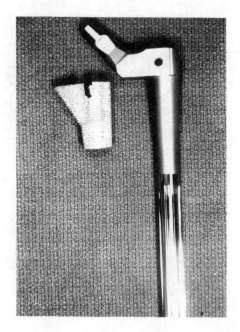

FIG. 5 -- S-ROM Modular Hip System.

RESULTS

IMPACT Modular Hip System

Eleven femoral stem systems were evaluated for the IMPACT Modular Hip System. Three stems survived 10 million cycles without failure for peak loads of 612 kgf, 625 kgf and 633 kgf (Table 1). The largest load applied to this design was 816 kgf.

In seven cases, stem failure occurred slightly proximal to the distal end of the metaphyseal component, within the metaphyseal/diaphyseal component taper and initiated across a lateral fretting surface (Fig. 6). In one case, the locking screw backed out causing cessation of the testing prior to stem fracture.

TABLE 1 -- IMPACT Modular Hip System results.

Peak Load Applied, kgf	Number of Cycles to Failure
816	24 600
765	68 900
625	312 600
663	867 900
714	2 019 600
689	2 392 300
653	5 079 900
638	9 234 300
612	10 000 000 (no failure)
625	10 000 000 (no failure)
633	10 000 000 (no failure)

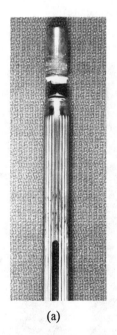
(a)

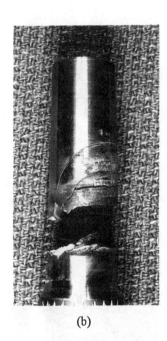
(b)

FIG. 6 -- Failed IMPACT Modular Hip System. (a) M-L view of a failed diaphyseal component. (b) A close-up antero-lateral view of the fracture site.

INFINITY Modular Hip System

Nine femoral stem systems were evaluated for the INFINITY Modular Hip System. Two stems survived 10 million cycles without failure for peak loads of 318 kgf and 409 kgf (Table 2). The largest load applied to this design was 590 kgf.

TABLE 2 -- INFINITY Modular Hip System results.

Peak Load Applied, kgf	Number of Cycles to Failure
443	213 300
590	222 900
500	232 200
431	234 300
454	240 400
477	478 600
386	8 259 200
318	10 000 000 (no failure)
409	10 000 000 (no failure)

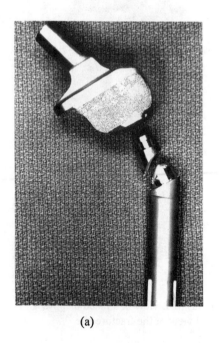
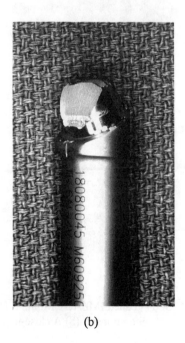

(a)   (b)

FIG. 7 -- Failed INFINITY Modular Hip System. (a) A-P view showing a failed device. (b) A close-up antero-medial view of the fracture site.

All cases of stem failure initiated across a lateral fretting surface at the mid-height of the trochanter/stem taper (Fig. 7).

RMHS Modular Hip System

Twelve femoral stem systems were evaluated for the RMHS Modular Hip System. Four stems survived 10 million cycles without failure for peak loads of 408 kgf, 612 kgf, 663 kgf and 714 kgf (Table 3). The largest load applied to this design was 918 kgf.

TABLE 3 -- RMHS Modular Hip System results.

Peak Load Applied, kgf	Number of Cycles to Failure
867	19 600
918	70 700
714	106 600
816	497 700
765	809 500
816	1 368 800
714	1 464 200
765	1 552 700
408	10 000 000 (no failure)
612	10 000 000 (no failure)
663	10 000 000 (no failure)
714	10 000 000 (no failure)

In this study, stem failure location was not consistent. Fracture initiated on the lateral aspect of the stem through the distal end of the sintered porous pad. This crack propagated through the pad attachment sites. While fretting was observed on the anterior pad/stem interface, it was not felt to be a contributory factor to failure (Fig. 8). Other locations included failure through the femoral neck and across the mid-stem where a change in curvature occurs. Because these failures did not initiate at metal-metal interfaces, fretting was not implicated as a contributor.

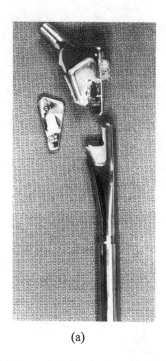

(a)

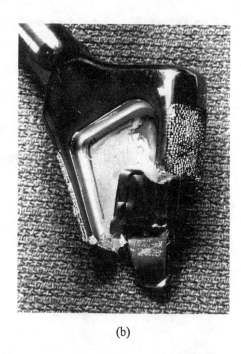

(b)

FIG. 8 -- Failed RMHS Modular Hip System. (a) A-P view showing a failed device. (b) A close-up antero-lateral view of the fracture site.

S-ROM Modular Hip System

Twelve femoral stem systems were evaluated for the S-ROM Modular Hip System. Three stems survived 10 million cycles without failure for peak loads of 454 kgf, 499 kgf and 568 kgf (Table 4). The largest load applied to this design was 681 kgf.

TABLE 4 -- S-ROM Modular Hip System results.

Peak Load Applied, kgf	Number of Cycles to Failure
499	121 500
613	125 800
658	143 900
579	178 800
590	238 000
636	248 700
568	331 700
681	602 000
522	7 409 700
454	10 000 000 (no failure)
499	10 000 000 (no failure)
568	10 000 000 (no failure)

All cases of stem failure occurred slightly proximal to the distal end of the sleeve, within the sleeve/stem taper and initiated across a lateral fretting surface (Fig. 9).

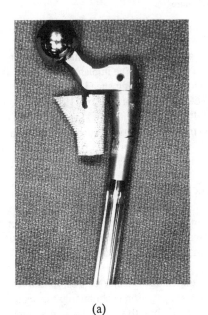
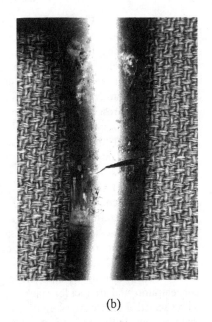

(a)   (b)

FIG. 9 -- Failed S-ROM Modular Hip System. (a) A-P view showing a failed device. (b) A close-up A-P view of the fracture site.

EVALUATION
Structural Fatigue Methodology
  Structural Fatigue Curve -- The characteristics of a structural fatigue curve are visualized in Fig. 10.

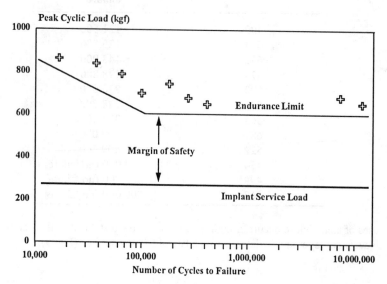

FIG. 10 -- Example of a structural fatigue curve.

In this study, the endurance limit is defined as the largest load at which 10 million, uninterrupted cycles occur without device failure. The value for the implant service load is dependent on patient weight and gait parameters including walking speed and stride length. For this study, a 74 kgf patient (male, age 60 years, height 173 cm [19]) was assumed with a resulting maximum joint force of 4 x body weight (296 kgf) [20]. The margin of safety serves as an indicator of implant structural integrity. Margins of safety are important in predicting implant longevity as population weight varies and unknown factors increase the implant service load (i.e., high activity level) or decrease the endurance limit (i.e., corrosion).

The structural fatigue curve is influenced by several parameters including stem geometry, neck length, material properties and surface preparation. Neck length is important as it determines the system's moment arm. Larger moment arms produce larger tensile bending stresses on the lateral side of the stem. When analyzing a structural fatigue curve, the moment arm or neck offset coupled with the applied load determines the severity of the loading environment.

Sites of fretting, notches due to porous coating and surface defects serve as stress concentrators and are foci for crack initiation. Crack propagation is commonly associated with oscillating tensile stress. In the case of the prosthetic hip, this translates into a crack that generally, initiates on the lateral side and propagates medially.

IMPACT Modular Hip System

The structural fatigue curve for the IMPACT system evaluated indicates an endurance limit 2.1 times the implant service load (Fig. 11).

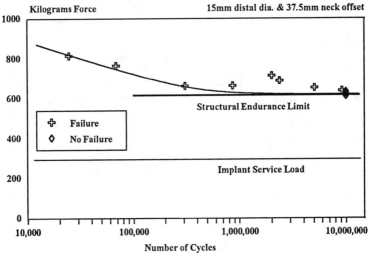

FIG. 11 -- Structural fatigue curve for IMPACT Modular Hip System.

INFINITY Modular Hip System

The structural fatigue curve for the INFINITY system evaluated indicates an endurance limit of 1.3 times the implant service load (Fig. 12).

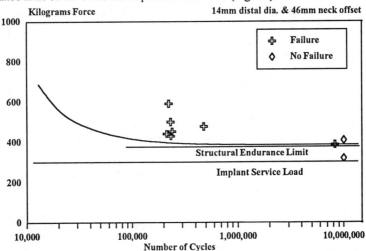

FIG. 12 -- Structural fatigue curve for INFINITY Modular Hip System.

RMHS Modular Hip System

The structural fatigue curve for the RMHS system evaluated indicated an endurance limit 2.3 times the implant service load (Fig. 13).

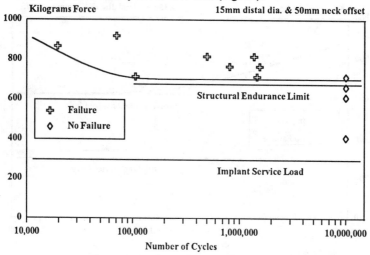

FIG. 13 -- Structural fatigue curve for RMHS Modular Hip System.

S-ROM Modular Hip System

The structural fatigue curve for the S-ROM system evaluated indicates an endurance limit 1.5 times the implant service load (Fig. 14).

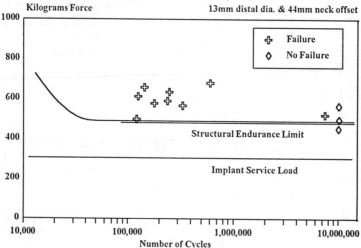

FIG. 14 -- Structural fatigue curve for S-ROM Modular Hip System.

In this study, the margin of safety for all of the design evaluated suggests that the fretting induced failure should not influence the device's longevity during *in vivo* service loading for a 74 kgf patient. As patient weight increases, the margin of safety will be reduced for this implant size.

DISCUSSION

The method described in this paper allows systems to be tested in a manner approximating *in vivo* support conditions. Clinical failure modes encountered with contemporary hip systems are predominantly manifested through the loss of proximal component support and require revision [1]. In this sense, structural failure of the component in the distal potting mode advocated in current ISO standards represents an unrealistic clinical loading scenario. Distal fixation prescribes failure location adjacent to the proximal edge of the potting material. In contrast, proximal mounting utilizes only the bone ingrowth/ongrowth surfaces for fixation and produces more realistic *in vivo* structural failures. Further, insistence on the utilization of distal potting methods precludes realistic structural support evaluations for composite, modular and monolithic stems of small size.

The development of a structural fatigue curve differs from a standard (S-N) fatigue curve in that the system as a whole is evaluated rather than individual components or test coupons. Once the baseline curve for a system has been established the influence of parameter variations, inclusive of manufacturing methodology and component sizing, can be studied with a smaller number of stems.

In this particular evaluation, an air environment was deliberately chosen in the recognition that testing frequencies between 10 Hz and 15 Hz precluded any short-term corrosion effects. In the longer *in vivo* view, however, one cannot overlook the potential degradation of structural integrity in a corrosive environment. The choice of an air environment, as well as, that of on-axis loading and neutral anteversion are presented here in an attempt to isolate the variables that influence fatigue failure. This methodology is sufficiently versatile to allow the inclusion of fluid submersion, off-axis loading and stem anteversion by design or pathology.

Although individual structural fatigue curves are of considerable value in assessing structural performance of a given system, they do not readily lend themselves to comparative analysis. For interdesign comparisons, a single patient anthropometry must be established inclusive of endosteal geometry, bone quality, neck offset and patient weight. The subsequent clinical selection of the optimal size for each design for this patient would enable the completion of a fatigue comparison.

CONCLUSION

A method of fatigue testing which incorporates proximal support and the effects of component interaction for modular femoral stems has been presented. It has been used to develop structural fatigue curves and endurance limits for four contemporary hip designs which serve, in this instance, as system examples of the application of this proximal support methodology. The results demonstrate that the *in vivo* structural integrity of these systems should not be compromised by the presence of metal-metal interconnections.

REFERENCES

[1]   Chandler, H., Clark, J., Murphy, S., McCarthy, J., Penenberg, B., Danylchuk, K., and Roehr, B., "Reconstruction of Major Segmental Loss of the Proximal Femur in Revision Total Hip Arthroplasty," Clinical Orthopaedics and Related Research, No. 298, January 1994, pp 67-74.

[2]   Gorski, J.M., "Modular Noncemented Total Hip Arthroplasty for Congenital Dislocation of the Hip: Case Report and Design Rationale," Clinical Orthopaedics and Related Research, No. 228, March 1988, pp 110-116.

[3]   Huckstep, C.M.G., "Stabilization and Prosthetic Replacement in Difficult Fractures and Bone Tumors," Clinical Orthopaedics and Related Research, No. 224, November 1987, pp 12-25.

[4]   Whiteside, L.A., Arima, J., White, S.E., Branam, L., and McCarthy, D.S., "Fixation of the Modular Total Hip Femoral Component in Cementless Total Hip Arthroplasty," Clinical Orthopaedics and Related Research, No. 298, January 1994, pp 184-190.

[5]   Bobyn, J.D., Tanzer, M., Krygier, J.J., Dujovne, A.R., and Brooks, E., "Concerns with Modularity in Total Hip Arthroplasty," Clinical Orthopaedics and Related Research, No. 298, January 1994, pp 27-36.

[6]   Collier, J.P., Surprenant, V.A., Jensen, M.S., and Mayor, M.B., "Corrosion at the Interface of Cobalt-Alloy Heads on Titanium-Alloy Stems," Clinical Orthopaedics and Related Research, No. 271, October 1991, pp 305-312.

[7]   Collier, J.P., Surprenant, V.A., Jensen, R.E., Mayor, M.B., and Surprenant, H.P., "Corrosion Between the Components of Modular Femoral Hip Prostheses," Journal of Bone and Joint Surgery, Vol. 74-B, No. 4, July 1992, pp 511-517.

[8]   Kummer, F.J. and Rose, R.M., "Corrosion of Titanium/Cobalt-Chromium Alloy Couples," Journal of Bone and Joint Surgery, Vol. 65-A, No. 8, October 1983, pp 1125-1126.

[9]   Lucas, L.C., Buchanan, R.A., and Lemons, J.E., "Investigations on the Galvanic Corrosion of Multialloy Total Hip Prostheses," Journal of Biomedical Material Research, Vol. 15, 1981, pp 731-747.

[10]   Mathiesen, E.B., Lindgren, J.U., Bloomgren, G.G.A., and Reinholt, F.P.O., "Corrosion of Modular Hip Prostheses," Journal of Bone and Joint Surgery, Vol. 73-B, No. 4, July 1991, pp 569-575.

[11]   Ohl, M.D., Whiteside, L.A., McCarthy, D.S., and White, S.E., "Torsional Fixation of a Modular Femoral Hip Component," Clinical Orthopaedics and Related Research, No. 287, February 1993, pp 135-141.

[12]   Pellicci, P.M. and Haas, S.B. "Disassembly of a Modular Femoral Component During Closed Reduction of the Dislocated Femoral Component," Journal of Bone and Joint Surgery, Vol. 72-A, No. 4, April 1990, pp 619-620.

[13]   Rand, J.A. and Chao, E.Y., Femoral Implant Neck Fracture Following Total Hip Arthroplasty," Clinical Orthopaedics and Related Research, No. 221, August 1987, pp 255-259.

[14]   Rostoker, W., Galante, J.O., and Lereim, P., "Evaluation of Couple/Crevice Corrosion by Prosthetic Alloys Under In Vivo Conditions," Journal of Biomedical Material Research, Vol. 12, 1978, pp 823-9.

[15]   Woolson, S.T., and Pottorff, G.T., " Disassembly of a Modular Femoral Prosthesis After Dislocation of the Femoral Component: A Case Report," Journal of Bone and Joint Surgery, Vol. 72-A, No. 4, April 1990, pp 624-625.

[16]   Postak, P.D., Polando, G., Pugh, J.W., and Greenwald, A.S., "A New Method of Fatigue Testing for Proximally Supported Femoral Stems," Scientific Exhibit, American Academy of Orthopaedic Surgeons Annual Meeting, Anaheim, CA, March 7 - 12, 1991.

[17]   Heim, C.S., Postak, P.D., and Greenwald, A.S., "Femoral Stem Fatigue Characteristics of Modular Hip Designs," Orthopaedic Transactions, Vol. 18, No. 4, 1994-1995, pp 1142-1143.

[18]   Heim, C.S., Postak, P.D., and Greenwald, A.S., "Femoral Stem Fatigue Characteristics of Modular Hip Designs - Series II," Orthopaedic Transactions Vol. 19, No. 2, 1995, pp 471-472.

[19]   Diem, K. and Lentner, C., Scientific Tables, Ciba-Geigy Limited, Switzerland, 1973, p 711.

[20]   Crowninshield, R.D., Johnston, R.C., Andrews, J.G., and Brand, R.A., "A Biomechanical Investigation of the Human Hip," Journal of Biomechanics, Vol. 11, No. 1/2, January 1978, pp 75-85.

Author Index

A

Abera, A., 189
Anthony, M. E., 85, 137

B

Bechtold, J. E., 114
Bhambri, S. K., 146
Bragdon, C. R., 33
Brown, S. A., 189
Buchanan, D. J., 199
Buckley, C. A., 157

C

Calès, B. J., 68
Cavallo, R. J., 5
Cooper, M. B., 85, 137

D

D'Onofrio, M., 189

F

Flemming, C., 189
Fosco, D. R., 199

G

Galante, J. O., 33
Gilbert, J. L., 33, 45, 157
Gilbertson, L. N., 146
Goldberg, J. R., 157
Goodman, S. B., 21
Greenwald, A. S., 226

H

Heim, C. S., 226
Holbrook, J. A., 85, 137
Huie, P., 21

J

Jacobs, J. J., 33, 45, 157

Jani, S. C., 211
Jasty, M., 33

K

Kirkpatrick, L. A., 94
Kovacs, P., 211
Kummer, F. J., 5
Kyle, R. F., 114

L

Lambert, R. D., 60, 104, 177, 211
Loch, D. A., 114

M

Maloney, W. J., 21
McLean, T. W., 60, 104, 177, 211

O

O'Connor, M., 21
Osthues, F. G., 127

P

Postak, P. D., 226

R

Rice, S. B., 33
Richter, H. G., 127

S

Salehi, A. B., 137
Sauer, W. L., 211
Schmidt, A. H., 114
Schurman, D. J., 21
Shea, J. J., 60
Sibley, R., 21
Song, Y., 21

U

Urban, R. M., 33

245

Subject Index

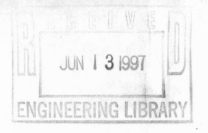